Acute nonlymphocytic leukaemia in adults

CLINICAL RESEARCH SERIES

The aim of this series is to draw attention to results of clinical research projects of interest to physicians in the field of internal medicine and related disciplines.
The editors hope that by reaching a wide audience, it will increase and facilitate practical application of recent findings.

Acute nonlymphocytic leukaemia in adults

Treatment and infection prevention

A.W. Dekker

1984
FORIS PUBLICATIONS
Dordrecht - Holland/Cinnaminson - U.S.A.

Published by:
Foris Publications Holland
P.O. Box 509
3300 AM Dordrecht, The Netherlands

Sole distributor for the U.S.A. and Canada:
Foris Publications U.S.A.
Cinnaminson N.J. 08077
U.S.A.

ISBN 90 6765 088 9

Printed in the Netherlands by ICG Printing, Dordrecht.

To my parents
For Yolanda

Contents

Introduction

Acute nonlymphocytic leukaemia (ANLL) is the most common type of acute leukaemia in adults. It is a serious disease which can only be treated with intensive cytotoxic chemotherapy adequately if optimal supportive care is available. This thesis deals with two subjects: (1) the analysis of the results obtained in patients with ANLL treated between 1977 and 1982, and (2) a study of the most effective and suitable regimen for the prevention of infections. Because infection is a major cause of death during remission induction treatment, studies of infection prevention in these patients are mandatory.

The first three chapters deal with the clinical aspects and results of treatment in patients with ANLL. Chapter 1 is a general introduction to the treatment of ANLL in adult patients with a review of the literature. In Chapter 2 a group of 114 patients with ANLL is analysed retrospectively and the results of remission induction therapy in 89 evaluable patients from this group are discussed. We observed a relatively high incidence of meningeal leukaemia in these patients. Because only few data were available about this difficult problem, a more extensive study was made of the clinical aspects of meningeal leukaemia and of the possibilities for prophylactic treatment (Chapter 3).

In Chapter 4 we discuss the possibilities of prevention of infections during remission induction treatment. The next three chapters describe the efficacy of three different regimens for selective decontamination. Chapter 5 presents the results of a controlled trial to ascertain the effect of prophylactic treatment with trimethoprim- sulfamethoxazole. In Chapter 6 the combination of trimethoprim-sulfamethoxazole plus colistin is evaluated. In Chapter 7 the results of two regimens for the prevention of infections are compared: colistin plus neomycin and colistin plus trimethoprim- sulfamethoxazole.

The general discussion (Chapter 8) includes some suggestions which might lead to improvement of the long term prognosis of ANLL.

CHAPTER 1

Chemotherapy and prognosis of acute nonlymphocytic leukaemia in adults

A review of the literature

INTRODUCTION

The initial objective of therapy in acute leukaemia is a complete remission, the achievement of which is a prerequisite for optimal palliation in the form of prolongation of symptom-free life and for maximizing the chance of cure (1). **Remission induction chemotherapy** is the therapeutic strategy using intensive cytotoxic drug combinations in order to achieve a complete remission which is commonly defined as a reduction of the number of leukaemic cells to very low levels (less than 5 percent of all nucleated cells in the bone marrow) with restoration of normal haematopoiesis (2,3,4,5). However, restoration of haematopoiesis occurs already with 2 logarithm reduction of leukaemic cell numbers i.e. a reduction of the leukaemic cell mass from 10^{11-12} to 10^{9-10} (6). The persistence of leukaemic cells in most patients who achieve complete remission is indicated by the high rate of relapse. The most common approach to prevent the recurrence of leukaemia has been the administration of chemotherapy to patients in remission. Three types of postremission chemotherapy are frequently distinguished: **consolidation chemotherapy**, using similarly high doses of drugs as used for remission induction, **maintenance chemotherapy**, using lower doses of the same or new drugs (7), and **intensification chemotherapy** involving high-dose chemotherapy with drugs that the patient has not received previously. A relatively new concept is the intensive **post-remission induction chemotherapy** combining consolidation therapy and intensification therapy with sequential non-cross-resistant drug combinations with the aim to maximize cytoreduction of residual leukaemic cells and to prevent the emergence of drug resistant cell lines (8,9,10). The following review will discuss the development of cytotoxic chemotherapy and the prognosis of acute nonlymphocytic leukaemia (ANLL) in adult patients. We use the term nonlymphocytic, alternative names are: nonlymphoblastic, myeloblastic, granulocytic, myelocytic, myeloid or myelogenous.

REMISSION INDUCTION CHEMOTHERAPY

Before 1948, there was no effective treatment for acute leukaemia. In 1953 the first results of the use of 6-mercaptopurine became available (11). The major advance in the treatment of ANLL was the introduction of cytosine arabinoside in 1966 (2) and of daunorubicin in 1967 (12). Cytosine arabinoside is a pyrimidine analogue that inhibits DNA synthesis by competitive inhibition of DNA polymerase; anthracycline antibiotics such as daunorubicin or adriamycine are thought to inhibit DNA replication by intercalation of base pairs (7). When cytosine arabinoside was used in a optimal schedule (200 mg/m^2/day for five days by continuous infusion) complete remission rates of 38% were achieved (13,14). Daunorubicin is probably the most effective single drug with a complete remission rate of 50% when doses to 60 mg/m^2/day for three days are used (5,15,16). Adriamycine (doxorubicin), a 14-hydroxyl derivate of daunorubicin, has not been studied on a large scale as single agent in the treatment of ANLL (5,17). There appears to be no advantage of adriamycine over daunorubicin (18,19), but the adriamycine excretion depends more on hepatic function, leading to prolonged plasma levels in patients with an impaired liver function (20,21,22).

A logical development was to combine active drugs in one schedule. Around 1970 clinical trials were initiated to study the efficacy of combination chemotherapy. The results from the first studies using cytosine arabinoside and thioguanine or 6-mercaptopurine were disappointing because too low doses had been used (23,24). In a subsequent study with increased doses (2.5 mg/kg/every 12 hours) of cytosine arabinoside and thioguanine in courses of 10 days a complete remission rate of 56% was achieved (25). The South West Oncology Group (SWOG) has conducted controlled trials to study cytosine arabinoside alone versus combination chemotherapy consisting of vincristine (O), cytosine arabinoside (A) and prednison (P) with or without the addition of cyclophosphamide (COAP) or daunorubicin (DOAP). There was only a slight improvement in response rate, 41% for combination chemotherapy (OAP, COAP, DOAP) versus 32% for cytosine arabinoside alone (14,26).

The combination of cytosine arabinoside with an anthracycline antibiotic is at present the most effective induction regimen (5,7). Before 1975, however, this combination yielded remission rates of not more than 50% (15,24,27,28). Some studies with more intensive schedules, in general combining three daily doses of daunorubicin (45 mg/m^2/day) with seven days courses of cytosine arabinoside (100 mg/m^2/day) "3 and 7" were more successful with remission rates over 60% (16,29,30). Although a large multicenter trial of the Cancer and Leukemia Group B confirmed the efficacy of this "3 and 7" regimen, as superior to the two days daunorubicin and five days cytosine arabinoside ("2 and 5") schedules, the remission rate was only

52% for the "3 and 7" regimen (31). In a later study it was found that the optimal daily dose of daunorubicin was 30 mg/m^2 for patients older than 60 years and 45 mg/m^2 for younger patients (19). It is not clear whether the addition of a third cytotoxic drug such as thioguanine to the combination of cytosine arabinoside and daunorubicin (TAD) has any value. Some studies achieved complete remission rates over 70% with this triple regimen (32,33,34,35,36), but other investigators found no improvement (37,38,39). At present a complete remission rate above 70% in adult patients with ANLL is exception rather than the rule (33,34) or is reported in studies with only a small number of patients (40,41) or with only young patients (10).

The crucial problem of remission induction treatment in patients with ANLL remains early death due to infection or bleeding (5,31,37,42,43). An intercurrent disease with subsequent death is a much more common cause of remission induction failure than drug resistant disease (44). The incidence of refractory leukaemia remained below 10% in recent studies (4,31,34,37, 44). Moreover the prognosis of patients with ANLL who fail to achieve a remission with intensive courses of cytosine arabinoside and an anthracycline antibiotic has improved since the introduction of amsacrine (AMSA)(45,46) and of high-dose cytosine arabinoside (47-51). New anthracycline antibiotics such as rubidazone, carminomycin and aclacinomycin (5) as well as amsacrine (1,52) and high-dose cytosine arabinoside (53) are not superior to cytosine arabinoside and daunorubicin or adriamycin as initial remission induction therapy.

POSTREMISSION CHEMOTHERAPY

The great variety of remission induction regimens with or without consolidation therapy makes it difficult to compare the data from maintenance schedules (5,7,8). One study may report the results of an "intensive consolidation" regimen, which in fact is less intensive than a "maintenance" regimen used by other investigators (10).

Controlled studies with a number of patients sufficient to determine the benefit of maintenance chemotherapy on the duration of remission are lacking. However, only those studies in which patients have been treated with consolidation courses or intensive maintenance courses have reported 10 to 20% of patients in continuous complete remission for more than five years (4,25,31,37,54). Treatment programs associated with a significant proportion of longterm survivors are the anthracycline-cytosine arabinoside and cytosine arabinoside regimens (55). Also, the best results of maintenance chemotherapy with respect to the median duration of complete remission are obtained if cytosine arabinoside and an anthracycline antibiotic are administered as part of the remission maintenance regimen (9,56). Recent studies using such type of maintenance therapy reported a median duration of remission of about 12 months (19,31,36). There is no evidence that maintenance chemotherapy will prolong the median duration of remission in patients who have received consolidation therapy (35). The results of studies using consolidation therapy without maintenance chemotherapy (34,35) or intensive maintenance chemotherapy without consolidation therapy (19,31,36) are comparable with respect to the median duration of remission and the proportion of continuous complete responders. A new development is the intensive post- remission induction chemotherapy consisting of sequential alternating courses with the most active antileukaemic agents at dose schedules equal to or greater than those given during induction. The aim of this approach is to maximize leukaemic cytoreduction, to minimize emergence of drug resistant cells and to eradicate minimal residual disease (8). The results with this intensive post-remission induction chemotherapy are promising especially in patients under 30 yrs of age (9,10), 50% will be remained in remission at 3 years (57). Unfortunately in older patients no plateau can be achieved (57) and 20% will still be in remission at 5 years (58). Also the toxicity in older patients leading to death during remission is high (at least 15%) with this therapy (58,59).

FACTORS PREDICTING RESPONSE TO THERAPY AND DURATION OF REMISSION

The identification of prognostic factors remains a point of controversy in the management of acute leukaemia. These factors are often related to a specific therapy or supportive care, and what is true in one institution is not necessarily true in another (1,60). Many prognostic factors of significance can be found after univariate analysis, but these factors can be interrelated. The use of multivariate analysis by a logistic regression model may resolve the relationship of each single factor and multiple factors to prognosis (1,61,62,63). The commonly accepted prognostic factors in predicting the probability of response are: age, morphologic cell type, initial white blood cell count, platelet count, secondary leukaemia and infection at admission.

The **age** of the patient is considered to be the most important prognostic factor (19,26,28,30,31,36,54,64,65), especially patients older than 50 years are susceptible to the complications of bone marrow failure and the toxic effects of antileukaemic drugs (19,43). There is no evidence that resistance to chemotherapy occurs more often in older patients. Although older age is an unfavourable factor for achieving complete remission it has no influence on the duration of remission (19,65,66). Response rates in older patients, however, have relatively improved in recent years (4,19,36,67) and in one single institution study older patients had the same remission rate as the younger patients (35).

The **morphologic characteristics** of the leukaemic cells in ANLL have occasionally been considered as a predictor for response. Acute promyelocytic leukaemia is often associated with excessive bleeding caused by disseminated intravascular coagulation and fibrinolysis (68) resulting in a higher incidence of early death from intracranial bleeding (69). Since the introduction of intensive chemotherapy (70) and extensive supportive care the prognosis has improved (54,70,72,73). Most investigators find a similar response rate and one recent study even supports an early report (70) in which promyelocytic leukaemia is associated with a prolonged remission (55). In a few studies, including also children, the duration of remission is short in acute monoblastic leukaemia (57,74). However, from recent large multicenter trials it is not possible to draw conclusions about the influence of a monoblastic cell type on the duration of remission because these studies had a very low incidence of this type of leukaemia (31,54). The presence of Auer rods at diagnosis may be a favourable prognostic factor for achieving complete remission (63,65,75) but this is not confirmed in another study (76). Studies using the FAB (French-American-British cooperative group) classification (77,78) are unable to show differences between the rate of remission, duration of remission and survival among these subtypes of ANLL (33,35,65, 76,79).

Peripheral **blood characteristics** such as haemoglobin level, platelet count and granulocyte count were previously thought to be independent factors influencing complete remission rate (61). In subsequent studies by the same group it was found that of these characteristics only a normal haemoglobin level at presentation was a favourable prognostic factor (63). This finding has not been confirmed, however, in a multicenter trial using the same remission induction therapy (54).

Hyperleucocytosis (> 100.000 leucocytes/μl) at presentation is often associated with a high incidence of early death from leucostasis complicated by haemorrhages in brain and lungs (80,81,82). The remission rate in patients with hyperleucocytosis is reported to be lower (54) or equal to that in patients with a lower white blood cell count (83,84). The duration of remission in patients with hyperleucocytosis is shortened (83,84).

Acute nonlymphocytic leukaemia occurring after prior exposure to cytotoxic chemotherapy with alkylating agents (85,86) or preceeded by a myelodysplastic (preleukaemic) disorder is associated with a low remission rate (5,7,87,88). The main reason for treatment failure is the severe and prolonged bone marrow aplasia after chemotherapy but also a higher incidence of resistance to chemotherapy is observed (67,89). Recently, Preisler et al. (90) have reported a high rate of complete remissions in ANLL secondary to cytotoxic therapy, using high doses of cytosine arabinoside alone for remission induction.

Ten years ago **infection at admission** was regarded as influencing unfavourably the chance of achieving remission (61). Since the introduction of broad spectrum antibiotics, however, this factor seems to have lost its prognostic significance (33,54,65,66).

It is not surprising that only few data are available of factors predicting long term survivorship (55,92), because there have been so few long term survivors (about 10%). The most important factor predicting long term survivorship is induction treatment using combination chemotherapy with cytosine arabinoside and an antracycline antibiotic, in which cytosine arabinoside seems to be the most important (55).

In conclusion studies dealing with prognostic factors have revealed inconsistent and controversial data. It is clear that prognostic factors which predict the probability of remission are quite different from the variables that have been discovered to predict duration of response. Also, these variables differ in their ability to detect the risk of recurrence at various intervals in the disease (1). At the present time commonly accepted prognostic factors should not be used to decide on the clinical management of acute leukaemia (5,93).

REFERENCES

1. Freireich EJ. Methods for evaluating response to treatment in adult acute leukemia. Blood Cells 9: 5-20, 1983.
2. Ellison RR, Holland JF, Weil M, Jacquillat C, Boiron M, Bernard J, Sawitsky A, Rosner F, Gussoff B, Silver RT, Karanas A, Cuttner J, Spurr CL, Hayes DM, Blom J, Leone LA, Haurani F, Kyle R, Hutchison JL, Jackson Forcier R, Moon JH. Arabinosyl cytosine: A useful agent in the treatment of acute leukemia in adults. Blood 32: 507-523, 1968.
3. Whittaker JA. Advances in the management of adult acute myelogenous leukaemia. Br Med J 281: 960-964, 1980.
4. Keating MJ, Smith TL, McCredie KB, Bodey GP, Hersh EM, Gutterman JU, Gehan E, Freireich EJ. A four-year experience with anthracycline, cytosine arabinoside, vincristine and prednisone combination chemotherapy in 325 adults with acute leukemia. Cancer 47: 2779-2788, 1981.
5. Foon KA, Gale RP. Controversies in the therapy of acute myelogenous leukemia. Am J Med 72: 963-979, 1982.
6. Frei E. Progress and perspectives in the chemotherapy of acute leukemia. Adv Chemother 2: 269-298, 1965.
7. Gale RP. Advances in the treatment of acute myelogenous leukemia. New Engl J Med 300: 1189-1199, 1979
8. Weinstein HJ, Mayer RJ, Rosenthal DS, Camitta BM, Coral FS, Nathan DG, Frei E III. Treatment of acute myelogenous leukemia in children and adults. New Engl J Med 303: 473-478, 1980.
9. Mayer RJ, Weinstein HJ, Coral FS, Rosenthal DS, Frei E III. The role of intensive postinduction chemotherapy in the management of patients with acute myelogenous leukemia. Cancer Treat Rep 66: 1455-1462, 1982.
10. Preisler HD. Therapy for patients with acute myelocytic leukemia who enter remission: Bone marrow transplantation or chemotherapy? Cancer Treat Rep 66: 1467-1473, 1982.

11. Gehan EA. Progress of therapy in acute leukemia 1948-1981: Randomized versus nonrandomized clinical trials. In: Controlled Clinical Trials 3. Elsevier Science Publishing Co. Inc., New York, pp. 199-207, 1982.
12. Boiron M, Jacquillat C, Weil M, Tanzer J, Levy D, Sultan C, Bernard J. Daunorubicin in the treatment of acute myelocytic leukaemia. The Lancet i: 330-333, 1969.
13. Southwest Oncology Group. Cytarabine for acute leukemia in adults. Effect of schedule on therapeutic response. Arch Intern Med 133: 251-259, 1974.
14. Bodey GP, Coltman CA, Freireich EJ, Bonnet JD, Gehan EA, Haut AB, Hewlett JS, McCredit KB, Saiki JH, Wilson HE. Chemotherapy of acute leukemia. Comparison of cytarabine alone and in combination with vincristine, prednisone, and cyclophosphamide. Arch Intern Med 133: 260-266, 1974.
15. Wiernik PH, Schimpff SC, Schiffer CA, Lichtenfeld JL, Aisner J, O'Connell MJ, Fortner C. Randomized clinical comparison of daunorubicin (NSC-82151) alone with a combination of daunorubicin, cytosine arabinoside (NSC-63878), 6-thioguanine (NSC-752), and pyrimethamine (NSC-3061) for the treatment of acute nonlymphocytic leukemia. Cancer Treat Rep 60: 41-53, 1976.
16. Weil M, Jacquillat CI, Gemon-Auclerc MF, Chastang CL, Israel V, Boiron M, Bernard J. Acute granulocytic leukemia. Treatment of the disease. Arch Intern Med 136: 1389-1395, 1976.
17. Wang JJ, Cortes E, Slinks LF et al. Therapeutic effect and toxicity of adriamycin in patients with neoplastic disease. Cancer 28: 837-843, 1972.
18. Wiernik PH. Sequential studies of daunorubicin and adriamycin in acute nonlymphocytic leukemia. Cancer Treat Rep 65 (Suppl. 4): 67-71, 1981.
19. Yates J, Glidewell O, Wiernik P, Cooper MR, Steinberg D, Dosik H, Levy R, Hoagland C, Menry P, Gottlieb A, Cornell C, Berenberg J, Hutchinson JL, Raich P, Nissen N, Ellison RR, Frelick R, James GW, Falkson G, Silver RT, Haurani F, Green M, Henderson E, Leone L, Holland JF. Cytosine arabinoside with daunorubicin or adriamycin for therapy of acute myelocytic leukemia: A CALGB study. Blood 60: 454-462, 1982.
20. Alberts DS, Bachur NR, Holtzman JL. The pharmacokinetics of daunomycin in man. Clin Pharmacol Ther 12: 96-104, 1971.
21. Benjamin RS, Riggs CE jr, Bachur NR. Pharmacokinetics and metabolism of adriamycin in man. Clin Pharmacol Ther 14: 592-600, 1973.
22. Benjamin RS, Wiernik PH, Bachur NR. Adriamycin chemotherapy-efficacy, safety, and pharmacologic basis of an intermittent single high-dosage schedule. Cancer 33: 19-27, 1974.
23. Gee TS, Yu K-P, Clarkson BD. Treatment of adult acute leukemia with arabinosylcytosine and thioguanine. Cancer 23: 1019-1032, 1969.
24. Carey RW, Ribas-Mundo M, Ellison RR, Glidewell O, Lee ST, Cuttner J, Levy RN, Silver R, Blom J, Haurani F, Spurr CL, Harley JB, Kyle R, Moon JH, Eagan RT, Holland JH. Comparative study of cytosine arabinoside therapy alone and combined with thioguanine, mercaptopurine, or daunorubicin in acute myelocytic leukemia. Cancer 36: 1560-1566, 1975.
25. Clarkson BD, Dowling MD, Gee TS, Cunningham IB, Burchenal JH. Treatment of acute leukemia in adults. Cancer 36: 775-795, 1975.
26. Coltman CA, Bodey GP, Hewlett JS, Haut A, Bickers J, Balcerzak SP, Costanzi JJ, Freireich EJ, McCredie KB, Groppe C, Smith TL, Gehan EA. Chemotherapy of acute leukemia. A comparison of vincristine, cytarabine, and prednisone alone and in combination with cyclophosphamide or daunorubicin. Arch Intern Med 138: 1342-1348, 1978.
27. Crowther D, Powles RL, Bateman CJT, Beard MEJ, Gaugi CL, Wrigley PFM, Malpas

JS, Hamilton Fairly GH, Bodley Scott R. Management of adult acute myelogenous leukaemia. Br Med J 1: 131-137, 1973.

28. Galton DAG, Bagshawe KD, Barkhan P, Bellingham AJ, Blackburn EK, Callender S, Delamore IW, Doll R, Durrant J, Fennelly JJ, Fraser ID, Hayhoe FJG, Hobbs JR, Innes J, Kay HEM, Marsh GW, McDonald GA, MacLennan ICM, Nelson MG, Peto R, Powles R, Roath OS, Roberts BE, Stuart J, Thompson RB, Wetherley-Mein G, Whittaker JA, Wiltshaw E. Chemotherapy of acute myeloid leukaemia in adults. Br J Cancer 39: 69-84, 1979.
29. Yates JW, Wallace HJ, Ellison RR. Cytosin arabinoside (NSC-63878) and daunorubicin (NSC-83142) therapy in acute nonlymphocytic leukemia. Cancer Chemother Rep 57: 485-491, 1973.
30. Preisler HD, Rustum Y, Henderson ES, Bjornsson S, Creaven PJ, Higby DJ, Freeman A, Gailani S, Naeher C. Treatment of acute nonlymphocytic leukemia: Use of anthracycline-cytosine arabinoside induction therapy and comparison of two maintenance regimens. Blood 53: 455-464, 1979.
31. Rai KR, Holland JF, Glidewell OJ, Weinberg V, Brunner K, Obrecht JP, Preisler HD, Nawabi IW, Prager D, Carey RW, Cooper MR, Haurani F, Hutchinson JL, Silver RT, Falkson G, Wiernik P, Hoagland HC, Bloomfield CD, James GW, Gottlieb A, Ramanan SV, Blom J, Nissen NI, Bank A, Ellison RR, Kung F, Henry P, McIntyre OR, Kaan SK. Treatment of acute myelocytic leukemia: A study by cancer and leukemia group B. Blood 58: 1203-1212, 1981.
32. Gale RP, Cline MJ for the UCLA Acute Leukemia Study Group. High remission-induction rate in acute myeloid leukaemia. The Lancet i: 497-499, 1977.
33. Gale RP, Foon KA, Cline MJ, Zighelboim J, and the UCLA Acute Leukemia Study Group. Intensive chemotherapy for acute myelogenous leukemia. Ann Intern Med 94: 753-757, 1981.
34. Urbanitz D, Buchner Th, Kamanabroo D, Hiddemann W, Schulte H, van de Loo J. Intensified remission induction therapy for acute nonlymphocytic leukemia (ANLL) treatment report on 60 patients. Blut 43: 129-133, 1981.
35. Foon KA, Zighelboim J, Yale C, Gale RP. Intensive chemotherapy is the treatment of choice for elderly patients with acute myelogenous leukemia. Blood 58, 467-470, 1981.
36. Buchner T, Urbanitz D, Emmerich B, Fischer JT, Fulle H-H, Heinecke A, Hossfeld DK, Koeppen KM, Labedzki L, Loffler H, Nowrousian MR, Pfreundschuh M, Pralle H, Ruhl H, Wendt F-C for the AML Cooperative Group. Multicentre study on intensified remission induction therapy for acute myeloid leukemia. Leuk Res 6: 827-831, 1982.
37. Glucksberg H, Cheever MA, Farewell VT, Fefer A, Sale GE, Thomas ED. High-dose combination chemotherapy for acute nonlymphoblastic leukemia in adults. Cancer 48: 1073-1081, 1981.
38. Armitage JO, Burns CP, Dick FR, Aunan SB, Slymen DJ. Results of aggressive chemotherapy for acute nonlymphoblastic leukemia in adults. Cancer Treat Rep 66: 1917-1924, 1982.
39. Henderson ES. Treatment of acute myelocytic leukemia (AML) (personal communication). 13th International Congress of chemotherapy, Vienna, 1983.
40. Rees JKH, Sandler RM, Challener J, Hayhoe FGJ. Treatment of acute myeloid leukaemia with a triple cytotoxic regime: DAT. Br J Cancer 36: 770-776, 1977.
41. Peterson BA, Bloomfield CD, Bosl GJ, Gibbs G, Malloy M. Intensive five-drug combination chemotherapy for adult acute non-lymphocytic leukemia. Cancer 46: 663-668, 1980.
42. Bodey GP, Rodriguez V, Chang H-Y, Narboni G. Fever and infection in leukemic patients. A study of 494 consecutive patients. Cancer 41: 1610-1622, 1978.

43. Estey EH, Keating MJ, McCredie KB, Bodey GP, Freireich EJ. Causes of initial remission induction failure in acute myelogenous leukemia. Blood 60: 309-315, 1982.
44. Preisler HD. Failure of remission induction in acute myelocytic leukemia. Med Pediatr Oncol 4: 275-276, 1978.
45. Legha SS, Keating MJ, Zander AR, McCredie KB, Bodey GP, Freireich EJ. 4'-(9-acridinylamino) methanesulfon-m-anisidide (AMSA): A new drug effective in the treatment of adult acute leukemia. Ann Intern Med 93: 17-21, 1980.
46. Lawrence HJ, Ries CA, Reynolds RD, Lewis JP, Koretz MM, Torti FM. AMSA - a promising new agent in refractory acute leukemia. Cancer Treat Rep 66: 1475-1478, 1982.
47. Rudnick SA, Cadman EC, Capizzi RL, Skeel RT, Bertino JR, McIntosh S. High dose cytosine arabinoside (HDARAC) in refractory acute leukemia. Cancer 44: 1189-1193, 1979.
48. Willemze R, Zwaan FE, Keuning JJ, Colpin G. Treatment of refractory acute leukaemia with high dose cytosine arabinoside. Br J Haematol 51: 497-504, 1982.
49. Willemze R, Zwaan FE, Colpin G, Keuning JJ. High dose cytosine arabinoside in the management of refractory acute leukaemia. Scand J Haematol 29: 141-146, 1982.
50. Herzig RH, Wolff SN, Lazarus HM, Phillips GL, Karanes C, Herzig GP. High-dose cytosine arabinoside therapy for refractory leukaemia. Blood 62: 361-369, 1983.
51. Willemze R, Fibbe WE, Zwaan FE. Experience with intermediate- and high-dose cytosine arabinoside in relapsed and refractory acute leukaemia. Neth J Med 26: 215-219, 1983.
52. Arlin ZA. 13th International Congress of Chemotherapy, Vienna. Part 207, 63-66 (abstract), 1983.
53. Spiers ASD. 3rd International Symposium on therapy of acute leukemias, Rome. p 44 (abstract), 1982.
54. McCredie KB, Gehan EA, Freireich EJ, Hewlett JS, Coltman CA, Hussein KK, Balcerzak SP, Chen TT. Management of adult acute leukemia. A southwest oncology group study. Cancer 52: 958-966, 1983.
55. Keating MJ, McCredie KB, Bodey GP, Smith TL, Gehan E, Freireich EJ. Improved prospects for long-term survival in adults with acute myelogenous leukemia. JAMA 248: 2481-2486, 1982.
56. Preisler HD. Acute myelocytic leukemia. In Leukemia, 4th edition, chapter 26. Gunz HW, Henderson ES, editors. Grune & Stratton, 1983.
57. Weinstein HJ, Mayer RJ, Rosenthal DS, Coral FS, Camitta BM, Gelber RD. Chemotherapy for acute myelogenous leukemia in children and adults: VAPA update. Blood 62: 315-319, 1983.
58. Weinstein HJ, Mayer RJ, Coral FS, Grier HE, Gelber RD, Rosenthal DA, Camitta BM, Frei III E. Remission duration in acute nonlymphocytic leukemia: practical and theoretical considerations. In: Minimal residual disease in acute leukemia. Lowenberg B, Hagenbeek A, eds., Martinus Nijhoff Publ., Boston, pp. 347-357, 1984.
59. Arlin Z. Is further intensification of treatment warranted in acute nonlymphoblastic leukemia? Cancer Treat Rep 67: 202-204, 1983.
60. Bloomfield CD, Arthur DC. Evaluation of leukemic cell chromosomes as a guide to therapy. Blood Cells 8: 501-518, 1982.
61. Gehan EA, Smith TL, Freireich EJ, Bodey G, Rodriguez V, Speer J, McCredie K. Prognostic factors in acute leukemia. Sem Oncol 3: 271-282, 1976.
62. Smith TL, Gehan EA, Keating MJ, Freireich EJ. Prediction of remission in adult acute leukemia. Development and testing of predictive models. Cancer 50: 466-472, 1982.
63. Keating MJ, Smith TL, Gehan EA, McCredie KB, Bodey GP, Freireich EJ. A prognostic factor analysis for use in development of predictive models for response in adult acute leukemia. Cancer 50: 457-465, 1982.

64. Bell R, Rohatiner AZS, Slevin ML, Ford JM, Dhaliwal HS, Henry G, Birkhead BG, Amess JAL, Malpas JS, Lister TA. Short-term treatment for acute myelogenous leukaemia. Br Med J 284: 1221-1224, 1982.
65. Passe S, Mike V, Mertelsmann R, Gee TS, Clarkson BD. Acute nonlymphoblastic leukemia. Prognostic factors in adults with long-term follow-up. Cancer 50: 1462-1471, 1982.
66. Keating MJ, Smith TL, Gehan EA, McCredie KB, Bodey GP, Spitzer G, Hersh E, Gutterman J, Freireich EJ. Factors related to length of complete remission in adult acute leukemia. Cancer 45: 2017-2029, 1980.
67. Keating MJ, McCredie KB, Benjamin RS, Bodey GP, Smith TL, Freireich EJ. Treatment of patients over 50 years of age with acute myelogenous leukemia with a combination of rubidazone and cytosine arabinoside, vincristine, and prednisone (ROAP). Blood 58: 584-591, 1981.
68. Gralnick HR, Abrell E. Studies of the procoagulant and fibrinolytic activity of promyelocytes in acute promyelocytic leukaemia. Br J Haematol 24: 89-99, 1973.
69. Jones ME, Saleem A. Acute promyelocytic leukemia. A review of literature. Am J Med 65: 673-677, 1978.
70. Bernard J, Weill M, Boiron M, Jacquillat C, Flandrin G, Gemon MF. Acute promyelocytic leukemia: Results of treatment by daunorubicin. Blood 41: 489-496, 1973.
71. Drapkin RT, Gee TS, Dowling MD, Arlin Z, McKenzie S, Kempin S, Clarkson B. Prophylactic heparin therapy in acute promyelocytic leukemia. Cancer 41: 2484-2490, 1978.
72. Collins AJ, Bloomfield CD, Peterson BA, McKenna RW, Edson JR. Acute promyelocytic leukemia. Management of the coagulopathy during daunorubicin- prednisone remission induction. Arch Intern Med 138: 1677-1680, 1978.
73. McKenna RW, Parkin J, Bloomfield CD, Sundberg RD, Brunning RD. Acute promyelocytic leukaemia: a study of 39 cases with identification of a hyperbasophilic microgranular variant. Br J Haematol 50: 201-214, 1982.
74. Tobelem G, Jacquillat C, Chastang C, Auclerc M-F, Lechevallier T, Weil M, Daniel M-T, Flandrin G, Harrousseau J-L, Schaison G, Boiron M, Bernard J. Acute monoblastic leukemia: A clinical and biological study of 74 cases. Blood 55: 71-76, 1980.
75. Zittoun R. 3rd International Symposium on therapy of acute leukemias. Rome, p 219 (abstract), 1982.
76. Sultan C, Deregnaucourt J, Ko JW, Imbert M, Ricard D'Agay MF, Gouault-Heilmann M, Brunn B. Distribution of 250 cases of acute myeloid leukaemia (AML) according to the FAB classification and response to therapy. Br J Haematol 47: 545-551, 1981.
77. Bennett JM, Catovsky D, Daniel M-T, Flandrin G, Galton DAG, Gralnick HR, Sultan C. Proposals for the classification of the acute leukaemias. Br J Haematol 33: 451-458, 1976.
78. Gralnick HR, Galton DAG, Catovsky D, Sultan C, Bennet JM. Classification of acute leukemia. Ann Intern Med 87: 740-753, 1977.
79. Mertelsmann R, Drapkin RL, Gee TS, Kempin S, Passe S, Thaler HT, Arlin Z, Dowling M, Dufour P, McKenzie S, To L, Comacho E, Oettgen HF, Burchenal JH, Clarkson B. Treatment of acute nonlymphocytic leukemia in adults: response to 2,2-anhydro-1- B-D-arabinofuranosyl-5-fluorocytosine and thioguanine on the L-12 protocol. Cancer 48: 2136-2142, 1981.
80. Freireich EJ, Thomas LB, Frei E III, Fritz RD, Forkner CE. A distinctive type of intracerebral hemorrhage associated with "blastic crisis" in patients with leukemia. Cancer 13: 146-154, 1960.
81. Harris AL. Leukostasis associated with blood transfusion in acute myeloid leukaemia. Br Med J 1: 1169-1171, 1978.

82. Reiffers J, Raynal F, Broustet A. Acute myeloblastic leukemia in elderly patients. Treatment and prognostic factors. Cancer 45: 2816-2820, 1980.
83. Vaughan WP, Kimball AW, Karp JE, Dragon LH, Burke PJ. Factors affecting survival of patients with acute myelocytic leukemia presenting with high Wbc counts. Cancer Treat Rep 65: 1007-1013, 1981.
84. Hug V, Keating M, McCredie K, Hester J, Bodey GP, Freireich EJ. Clinical course and response to treatment of patients with acute myelogenous leukemia presenting with a high leukocyte count. Cancer 52: 773-779, 1983.
85. Rosner F, Grunwald HW. Cytotoxic drugs and leukaemogenesis. Clinics in Haematology 3: 663-681, 1980.
86. Boice JD Jr, Greene MH, Killen JY Jr, Ellenberg SS, Keehn RJ, McFadden E, Chen TT, Fraumeni JF Jr. Leukemia and preleukemia after adjuvant treatment of gastrointestinal cancer with semustine (Methyl-CCNU). New Engl J Med 309: 1079-1084, 1983.
87. Koeffler HP, Golde DW. Human preleukemia. Ann Intern Med 93: 347-353, 1980.
88. Bennett JM, Catovsky D, Daniel MT, Flandrin G, Galton DAG, Gralnick HR, Sultan C, the French- American-British (FAB) Co-operative group. Proposals for the classification of the myelodysplastic syndromes. Br J Haematol 51: 189-199, 1982.
89. Rosner F, Grunwald H. Acute leukemia associated with chemotherapy. Arch Intern Med 143: 1322-1323, 1983.
90. Preisler HD, Early AP, Raza A, Vlahides G, Marinello MJ, Stein AM, Browman G. Therapy of secondary acute nonlymphocytic leukemia with cytarabine. New Engl J Med 308: 21-22, 1983.
91. Lister TA, Whitehouse JMA, Oliver RTD, Bell R, Johnson SAN, Wrigley PFM, Ford JM, Cullen MH, Gregory W, Paxton AM, Malpas JS. Chemotherapy and immunotherapy for acute myelogenous leukemia. Cancer 46: 2142-2148, 1980.
92. Whittaker JA, Reizenstein P, Callender ST, Cornwell GG, Delamore IW, Gale RP, Gobbi M, Jacobs P, Lantz B, Maiolo AT, Rees JKH, van Slyck EJ, Vu Van H. Long survival in acute myelogenous leukaemia: an international collaborative study. Br Med J 282: 692-695, 1981.
93. Brandman J, Bukowski RM, Greenstreet R, Hewlett JS, Hoffman GC. Prognostic factors affecting remission, remission duration, and survival in adult acute nonlymphocytic leukemia. Cancer 44: 1062-1065, 1979.

CHAPTER 2

The management of acute nonlymphocytic leukaemia in adults

Evaluation of the results in a non-selected group of 114 patients

A.W. Dekker, J.J. Sixma and K. Punt

Dept. of Haematology, University Hospital Utrecht, The Netherlands

SUMMARY

A retrospective analysis was made of all patients (114) who presented with acute nonlymphocytic leukaemia (ANLL) between February 1977 and December 1981. Five patients died before chemotherapy and in 10 patients induction therapy was contraindicated. Seven patients with secondary leukaemia were treated, no remission being achieved. A group of 89 evaluable patients with de novo ANLL was further analysed for response to induction treatment (doxorubicin, vincristine and cytosine arabinoside). The complete remission rate of this group was 48 per cent. There was a significant difference in remission rate, however, between patients under and above the age of 50 (66 per cent and 29 per cent, respectively; $p < 0.001$), and between patients with more or less than 100×10^9 leukaemic cells per liter (20 per cent and 54 per cent, respectively; $p < 0.01$). The remission rate was not different in the FAB subclasses and was not influenced by the presence or absence of infection at admission. The median survival time for complete responders was 20 months. The implications and some possible ways to improve them are discussed.

INTRODUCTION

In the past 15 years significant advances have been made in the treatment of adult acute nonlymphocytic leukaemia (ANLL). They have recently been reviewed in several articles (1,2) and also in this Journal (3,4). The introduction in 1966 of cytosine arabinoside opened a new era in chemotherapy for ANLL. If used as a single agent it induces complete remission, which is a prerequisite for prolonged survival, in about 25 per cent of cases (1,2). More recently, anthracyclines (daunorubicin or doxorubicin) have been combined with cytosine arabinoside for induction therapy, which has increased the remission rate to 50-80 per cent. The results of recent clinical trials (5-7) suggest that parameters such as age, infection at presentation, initial blast cell count and morphological subclass seem to be less important prognostic factors in relation to response rate than was previously thought (8,9). Interpretation of results is not always easy, especially in studies with a small number of patients or with a selected group of patients.

The purpose of this retrospective study is to evaluate all patients with ANLL admitted consecutively to our hospital between February 1977 and December 1981, because in this period the same induction treatment (including cytosine arabinoside and doxorubicin) was given to all suitable patients. A comprehensive report on 114 patients is presented, and prognostic factors such as age and hyperleucocytosis are discussed in detail.

PATIENTS AND METHODS

Patients

Between February 1977 and December 1981 a total of 114 adult patients with previously untreated ANLL were admitted to our hospital. The diagnosis was made by examination of pretreatment smears of blood and of bone marrow aspirates after conventional and cytochemical staining, and the cases were classified according to the French American British (FAB) system (10,11). The slides were reviewed by the Leukaemia Cytomorphology Committee of the Dutch Study Group for onco-haematological diseases in adults (HOVON).

Fifteen patients were excluded from evaluation: 5 died before treatment was started and in 10 patients remission induction therapy was not considered in view of severe complicating factors at presentation. Eighty- nine patients were fully evaluable. Ten other patients presented with secondary leukaemia, 6 after a dysmyelopoietic syndrome and 4 after treatment with alkylating agents for a previous malignancy; they were evaluated separately.

Induction and maintenance therapy

The remission induction treatment consisted of doxorubicin 50 mg/m^2 intravenously on day 1, vincristine 1 mg/m^2 i.v. on day 2 and cytosine arabinoside 80 mg/m^2 i.v. every 12 hours on days 3 to 8 (12). A second course was given 15 days after completion of the first course, but a longer interval was taken if at that time the marrow was still aplastic with less than 10 per cent leukaemic cells. No consolidation treatment was given; most patients younger than 65 years, however, received a second course if complete remission was already achieved after one course. No central nervous system prophylaxis was applied. Once a complete remission was achieved, maintenance chemotherapy was instituted and continued for 3 years at most. The weekly maintenance chemotherapy consisted of 6-thioguanine 2 mg/kg orally on four consecutive days, followed by cytosine arabinoside 1.5 mg/kg on the fifth day (13). Every 3 months a control bone marrow aspirate was obtained.

Supportive therapy

Transfusions of red blood cells and platelets were given when required. The haemoglobin level was maintained above 6 mmol/l. Random donor platelet concentrates were administered to maintain a platelet count above $10 \times 10^9/l$. Human leucocyte antigen (HLA)-matched platelets, if available, were given to patients refractory to random platelets. Patients were accommodated in single or double rooms or in a 6-bed ward. Twenty-six patients received trimethoprim- sulfamethoxazole (14) to prevent infection; 16 patients were treated with trimethoprim-sulfamethoxazole plus colistin. All patients with suspected infections or fever were given i.v. gentamicin (3 mg/kg daily, divided into three doses) and cephalothin (4×1.5 g daily). Only one patient was given granulocyte transfusions. All patients received allopurinol (300 mg daily). When the initial serum uric acid was increased, a high alkaline urine output was maintained during the first days of induction therapy with sodium bicarbonate 1.4%, 2000 ml i.v. in 24 hours.

Data analysis

Applying the criteria for evaluating response as formulated by the Cancer and Leukemia Group B (CALGB), a complete remission was defined as bone marrow containing less than 5 per cent leukaemic cells in the presence of a peripheral granulocyte count above 1.5×10^9 cells/l, a platelet count above $100 \times 10^9/l$ and no other evidence of leukaemia (15). In partial remission the bone marrow contained more than 5 per cent but less than 25 per cent leukaemic cells. A relapse was diagnosed at the re-appearance of more than 5 per cent leukaemic cells in the bone marrow or when extramedullary localizations developed.

The Kaplan-Meier method (16) was used to obtain the predictive survival and remission duration curves, calculated as of lst March 1982, with survival times measured from the date of diagnosis, and remission duration from the date of complete haemotological remission to the date of relapse. Comparison of responders with non-responders in different groups of patients was performed by chi-square analysis with Yates correction.

RESULTS

The median age and median survival of subgroups of 114 patients are presented in table 1. Five patients died before receiving any therapy. Poor survival was observed when induction treatment was contraindicated. Seven patients with secondary leukaemia were given induction therapy, but no complete remission was attained. Eighty-nine evaluable patients with ANLL were further analysed.

Remission induction

Patient characteristics and response to therapy are summarized in table 2. Of 89 patients, 41 were men and 48 women. The median age was 49 years (range 15 to 79 years); 47 per cent of these patients were over 50 years of age. Forty-three patients (48 per cent) achieved a complete remission, 46 were failures (52 per cent) including 6 patients with a partial remission (7 per cent) and 9 patients who died during the first days of treatment. The complete remission rate was independent of sex, hepato- and/or splenomegaly and the presence or absence of infection at the time of admission. The outcome of induction treatment was poor in patients over 50 years of age; 12 out of 42 (29 per cent) versus 31 out of 47 patients (66 per cent) younger than 50 years achieved a complete remission ($p < 0.001$). Hyperleucocytosis (defined as more than 100×10^9 leukaemic cells per l blood) was also a bad prognostic factor ($p < 0.01$). The remission rate was not influenced by the FAB subclasses, the number of patients with promyelocytic leukaemia (M_3) was too small for conclusions (table 3).

Table 1. Survival of 114 patients with acute nonlympocytic leukaemia (ANLL)

	Number		Median age (yrs)	Median survival (months)
De novo ANLL	104			
death before start of therapy		5	67	-
chemotherapy contraindicated		10	66	2
given induction therapy		89	49	8
complete responders		43	43	20
failures		46	62	1.5
Secondary ANLL	10		61	1
Total	114			

Table 2. Pretreatment characteristics and response rates of evaluable patients with acute nonlymphocytic leukaemia

Characteristic	Number of patients	Complete responders	(%)
Total	89	43	(48)
Age (yrs)			
≥ 50	42	12*	(29)
< 50	47	31*	(66)
Sex			
female	48	25	(52)
male	41	18	(44)
Infection or fever at admission	53	23 NS	(43)
No infection or fever at admission	36	20 NS	(56)
Hepato- and/or splenomegaly	8	5	(63)
Leucocyte count			
> 100,000/µl	15	3**	(20)
< 100,000/µl	74	40**	(54)

* $p < 0.001$, $\chi^2 = 13.96$.
** $p < 0.01$, $\chi^2 = 7.24$
NS: not significant.

The mean number of treatment courses was 1.9; 15 patients (35 per cent) achieved a complete remission after one course, 18 patients (42 per cent) after two courses and 10 after three courses (23 per cent). Thirty-five patients died during the induction period (table 4), including 7 patients (8 per cent) with refractory leukaemia, arbitrarily defined when after two courses of chemotherapy the bone marrow still contained more than 50 per cent blasts and/or when blast cells were present in the peripheral blood.

Table 3. FAB classification and response to therapy

Morphology	Number of patients	Complete responders	(%)
M1	16	7	(44)
M2	25	13	(52)
M3	6*	2	-
M4	27	12	(44)
M5	13	9	(69)
M6	1*	0	-
unclassifiable	1*	0	-

* Groups too small for conclusions.

Table 4. Causes of death during induction treatment

Infection	16
Haemorrhage	8
Combination	9
Others	2
Total	35

Remission duration and survival

The median remission duration was 8 months and the median survival of the complete responders was 20 months (figs. 1 and 2). The median survival of the entire group was 8 months. In spite of a two-year survival of 35 per cent of the complete responders, only one patient in this group remained free from disease for more than three years. The median survival of non-responders, including the patients who died during the first days, was less than 2 months (fig.2). The survival of 6 partial responders varied from 5 to 33 months (median survival 12 months). After achieving remission, no difference was found in remission duration between patients younger or older than 50 years (data not shown).

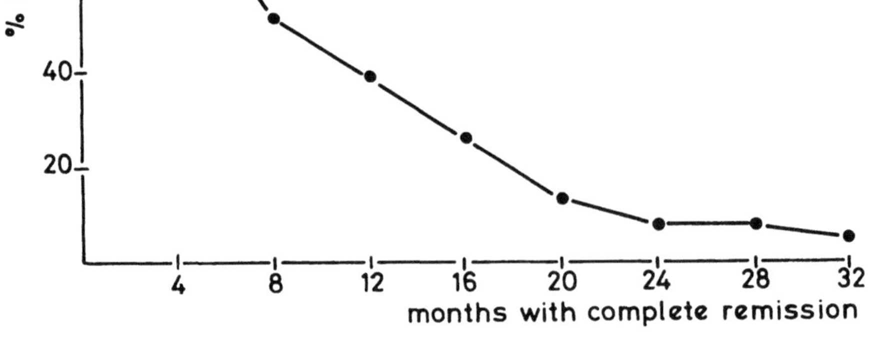

Figure 1. Actuarial curve of remission duration in 43 patients with ANLL.

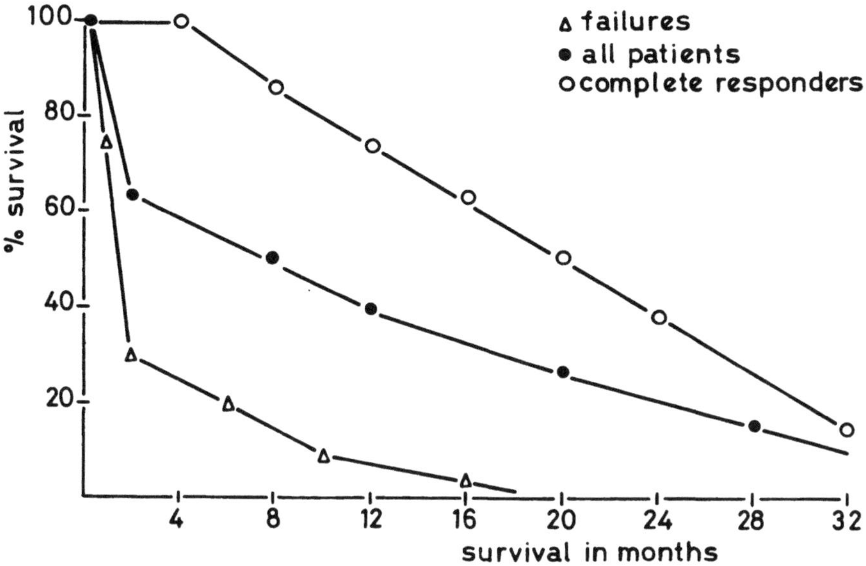

Figure 2. Actuarial survival of 89 evaluable patients with ANLL after institution of induction chemotherapy.

Twenty-four of the 30 patients with a haematological relapse were treated with another scheme of induction therapy, usually 6-thioguanine, cytosine arabinoside and daunorubicin (17) or doxorubicin with large doses of cytosine arabinoside. With this more intensive induction treatment, 12 patients (50 per cent) attained a second complete remission with a median duration of 3.5 months. Six patients with a meningeal relapse (14 per cent) were treated with intrathecal methotrexate or cytosine arabinoside combined with cranial irradiation. Only the three patients who showed no evidence of a concurrent haematological relapse achieved a remission.

Toxicity

In nearly all cases bone marrow aplasia developed within 7 days of completing induction chemotherapy. The mean number of days with a granulocyte count of less than 0.1×10^9/l during the total induction period was 24 days. The fever incidence during these days with profound granulocytopenia was 42 per cent. Thirty-five patients died during induction treatment, infection being the most common cause of death (table 4). Nine patients died during the first days of induction treatment; the most common causes were hyperleucocytosis with leucostasis (6 patients) and intravascular coagulation in promyelocytic leukaemia (3 patients).

DISCUSSION

The complete remission rate of the entire group of 89 evaluable patients with ANLL (secondary leukaemia excluded) was 48 per cent, with a median survival of 20 months in the complete responders versus 8 months in the entire group. The complete response rate was significantly higher in patients younger than 50 years (66 per cent) than in older patients (29 per cent). Studies by other groups of large numbers of patients have reported response rates of 32-66 per cent (6,7,9,18-24). With a few exceptions (7) complete remission rates of more than 60 per cent are related to studies of small numbers of patients (25-27) or of younger patients (12,28). A good example of how small numbers may lead to falsely optimistic views is our own experience in 1979, when the remission rate was 16 out of 20 patients (80 per cent).

Our observation that the percentage of patients who achieve a remission declines considerably with increasing age is in agreement with the experience of most authors (8,9,18,20-23). In our opinion, however, age alone should never be decisive in determining the feasibility of induction therapy, because survival is closely related to achieving complete remission. The present use of more intensive regimens with complete remission rates of 59-77 per cent after one course of chemotherapy (7,26,29), made possible by the progress in supportive treatment such as infection prevention by selective decontamination (14,30) and single-donor platelet transfusion (31), has substantially improved the prognosis in all age groups, including older patients (7,26,29,32,33). In these patients, too, provided they are in an otherwise good condition, early induction treatment can prevent death from infection or haemorrhage by limiting the period of bone marrow aplasia.

Patients with hyperleucocytosis (above 100×10^9 leukaemic cells/l) are at risk of early death from sludging and proliferation of blast cells in small vessels and capillary beds, with secondary tissue invasion and haemorrhage (leucostasis) (27,34-36). We had the same experience: 6 out of 9 patients who died during the first days of induction treatment suffered from hyperleucocytosis. The results in these patients may improve by rapid cytoreduction by leukapheresis (37-39), transfusion of large numbers of platelets (36) and avoidance of red blood cell transfusions which lead to an increase in viscosity (34), combined with promptly instituted chemotherapy.

The improvement in the results of induction treatment does not apply to therapy-linked leukaemia or leukaemia after a preleukaemic phase. No complete response was observed in our 7 treated patients with secondary leukaemia. The literature (1,22) also reports remission rates of less than 10 per cent. The decision whether or not to give such patients induction treatment, especially at an older age, remains controversial.

The incidence of central nervous system leukaemia (14 per cent) as a consequence of meningeal infiltration seems to be rather high. However, a 10-20 per cent incidence of clinically overt central nervous system leukaemia in ANLL has regularly been reported (1,2,6,23,40,41). Although prophylactic cranial irradiation and/or intrathecal chemotherapy are probably effective in preventing meningeal leukaemia (7,32), this approach has not prolonged the duration of systemic remission. For the time being central nervous system prophylaxis should therefore not be routinely recommended (2,7).

In spite of a two-year survival of 35 per cent of the complete responders, only one patient has remained free from disease after more than three years. Other centres have reported a 3 to 5-year (predictive) disease-free survival of 10 to 20 per cent (6,7,21-24,42). The reason for this discrepancy is obscure, as are the factors contributing to prolonged survival (43). Whether long-term survivors have been cured is a matter of speculation; relapses do still occur after 5 years' remission. Most patients relapse because they have some residual leukaemic cells, which probably begin to multiply as soon as induction treatment is discontinued. The significance of consolidation, intensification and maintenance chemotherapy in the prolongation of remission in these patients is still not clear (1,2,7,20,22-24,28). Another approach to eliminate residual leukaemia may be 'conditioning' with supralethal chemotherapy plus whole-body irradiation, followed by 'rescue' (transplantation) with donor or autologous bone marrow.

For the small group of patients in first remission who are under 40 and have an HLA-matched sibling willing to act as donor, intensive chemotherapy followed by allogeneic bone marrow transplantation should be seriously considered (4,44-46). Morbidity and mortality of this treatment are still high, however. A similar programme using autologous bone marrow transplantation is tolerated much better, but little is known of the long-term results. In our hospital such a programme has recently been started for patients with other malignancies. We intend to extend it to patients with ANLL in first remission and below the age of 50, in order to see whether disease-free survival can be prolonged.

ACKNOWLEDGEMENTS

We thank ms C.C. Bos for her expert technical assistance and ms A. Beyer for her secretarial assistance.

REFERENCES

1. Gale RP. Advances in the treatment of acute myelogenous leukemia. N Engl J Med 1979; 300: 1189-1199.
2. Whittaker JA. Advances in the management of adult acute myelogenous leukaemia. Br Med J 1980; I: 960-964.

3. Mulder NH. Therapy of acute leukaemia in adults. Neth J Med 1981; 24: 133-135.
4. Zwaan FE, Jansen J. Acute leukaemia, perspectives in diagnosis and treatment. Neth J Med 1981; 24: 190-194.
5. Brandman J, Bukowski RM, Greenstreet R, et al. Prognostic factors affecting remission, remission duration, and survival in adult acute nonlymphocytic leukemia. Cancer 1979; 44: 1062-1065.
6. Lister TA, Whitehouse JMA, Oliver RTD, et al. Chemotherapy and immunotherapy for acute myelogenous leukemia. Cancer 1980; 46: 2142-2148.
7. Gale RP, Foon KA, Cline MJ, et al. Intensive chemotherapy for acute myelogenous leukemia. Ann Intern Med 1981; 94: 753-757.
8. Gehan EA, Smith TL, Freireich EJ, et al. Prognostic factors in acute leukemia. Semin Oncol 1976; 3: 271-282.
9. Cuckle H, Galton DAG, Peto R. Chemotherapy of acute myeloid leukaemia in adults. Br J Cancer 1979; 39: 69-86.
10. Bennett JM, Catovsky D, Daniel MT, et al. Proposals for the classification of the acute leukaemias. Br J Haematol 1976; 33: 451-458.
11. Gralnick HR, Galton DAG, Catovsky D, et al. Classification of acute leukemia. Ann Intern Med 1977; 87: 740-753.
12. Mathe G, Misset JL, Pouillart P, et al. Remission induction in acute lymphoid and acute myeloid leukaemias. Lancet 1976; I: 1130-1131.
13. Peterson BA, Bloomfield CD. Prolonged maintained remissions of adult acute nonlymphocytic leukaemia. Lancet 1977; II: 158-160.
14. Dekker AW, Rozenberg-Arska M, Sixma JJ, Verhoef J. Prevention of infection by trimethoprim- sulfamethoxazole plus amphotericin B in patients with acute nonlymphocytic leukaemia. Ann Intern Med 1981; 95: 555-559.
15. Ellison RR, Holland JF, Weil M, et al. Arabinosyl cytosine: a useful agent in the treatment of acute leukemia in adults. Blood 1968; 32: 507-523.
16. Kaplan EL. Meier P. Non-parametric estimation from incomplete observations. Am Stat Assoc J 1958; 53: 457-481.
17. Gale RP, Cline MJ. High remission-induction rate in acute myeloid leukaemia. Lancet 1977; I: 497-499.
18. Willemze R, Den Ottolander GJ, Heering KJ, et al. Behandeling van acute myeloide leukemie bij volwassenen: een verantwoording over de jaren 1968 t/m 1975. Ned T Geneesk 1977; 121: 1843-1847.
19. Storms GEMG, Burghouts J, Haanen C. The favourable effect of immunotherapy on survival and the achievement of a second remission in acute myeloid leukaemia. Neth J Med 1980; 23: 54-58.
20. Preisler HD, Rustum Y, Henderson ES, et al. Treatment of acute nonlymphocytic leukemia: use of anthracycline-cytosine arabinoside induction therapy and comparison of two maintenance regimens. Blood 1979; 54: 455-464.
21. Rai KR, Holland JF, Glidewell OJ, et al. Treatment of acute myelocytic leukemia: a study by cancer and leukemia group B. Blood 1981; 58: 1203-1212.
22. Keating MJ, Smith TL, McCredie KB, et al. A four-year experience with anthracycline, cytosine arabinoside, vincristine and prednisone combination chemotherapy in 325 adults with acute leukemia. Cancer 1981; 47: 2779-2788.
23. Glucksberg H, Cheever MA, Farawell VT, et al. High-dose combination chemotherapy for acute nonlymphoblastic leukemia in adults. Cancer 1981; 48: 1073-1081.
24. Mertelsmann R, Drapkin RL, Gee TS, et al. Treatment of acute nonlymphocytic leukemia in adults: reponse to 2,2-anhydro-1-B-D- arabinofuranosyl- 5-fluorocytosine and thioguanine on the L-12 protocol. Cancer 1981; 48: 2136-2142.
25. Rees JKH, Sandler RM, Challener J, Hayhoe FGJ. Treatment of acute myeloid leukaemia with a triple cytotoxic regimen; DAT. Br J Cancer 1977; 36: 770-776.

26. Peterson BA, Bloomfield CD, Bosl GL, et al. Intensive five-drug combination chemotherapy for adult nonlymphocytic leukemia. Cancer 1980; 46: 663-668.
27. Reiffers J, Raynal F, Broustet A. Acute myeloblastic leukemia in elderly patients. Cancer 1980; 45: 2816-2820.
28. Weinstein HJ, Mayer RJ, Rosenthal DS, et al. Treatment of acute myelogenous leukemia in children and adults. N Engl J Med 1980; 303: 473-478.
29. Keating MJ, McCredie KB, Benjamin RS, et al. Treatment of patients over 50 years of age with acute myelogenous leukemia with a combination of rubidazone and cytosine arabinoside, vincristine and prednisone (ROAP). Blood 1981; 58: 584-591.
30. Sleyfer DT, Mulder NH, De Vries-Hospers HG, et al. Infection prevention of granulocytopenic patients by selective decontamination of digestive tract. Eur J Cancer 1980; 16: 859-869.
31. Sintnicolaas K, Vriezendorp HM, Sizoo W, et al. Delayed alloimmunisation by random single donor platelet transfusions. Lancet 1981; I: 750-753.
32. De Vries EGE, Mulder NH, Houwen B. Absence of the influence of age on remission rate and duration of remission in a group of thirty-four patients with acute myeloid leukaemia. Neth J Med 1980; 23: 241-245.
33. Foon KA, Zighelboim J, Yale C, Gale RP. Intensive chemotherapy is the treatment of choice for elderly patients with acute myelogenous leukemia. Blood 1981; 58: 467-470.
34. Harris AL. Leukostasis associated with blood transfusion in acute myeloid leukaemia. Br Med J 1978; I: 1169-1171.
35. Vernant JP, Brun B, Mannoni P, et al. Respiratory distress of hyperleukocytic granulocytic leukemias. Cancer 1979; 44: 264-268.
36. Vaughan WP, Kimball AW, Kapr JE, et al. Factors affecting survival of patients with acute myelocytic leukemia presenting with high Wbc counts. Cancer Treat Rep 1981; 65: 1007-1013.
37. Eisenstadt RS, Berkman EM. Rapid cytoreduction in acute leukemia. Transfusion 1978; 18: 113-115.
38. Lane TA. Continuous-flow leukapheresis for rapid cytoreduction in leukemia. Transfusion 1980; 20: 2017-2029.
39. Karp DD, Beck R, Cornell CJ. Chronic granulocytic leukemia with respiratory distress: efficacy of emergency leukapheresis. Arch Intern Med 1981; 141: 1353-1354.
40. Law IP, Blom J. Adult acute leukemia. Cancer 1977; 40: 1304-1306.
41. Meyer RJ, Ferreira PPC, Cuttner, et al. Central nervous system involvement at presentation in acute granulocytic leukemia. Am J Med 1980; 68: 691-694.
42. Weil M, Jacquillat CI, Gemon-Aucler MF, et al. Acute granulocytic leukemia. Arch Intern Med 1976; 136: 1389-1395.
43. Whittaker JA, Reizenstein I, Callender ST, et al. Long survival in acute myelogenous leukaemia: an international collaborative study. Br Med J 1981; II: 692-695.
44. Thomas ED, Buckner CD, Clift RA, et al. Marrow transplantation for acute non-lymphoblastic leukemia in first remission. N Engl J Med 1979; 301: 597-599.
45. Blume KG, Beutler E, Bross KJ, et al. Bone-marrow ablation and allogeneic marrow transplantation in acute leukemia. New Engl J Med 1980; 302: 1041-1046.
46. Powles RL, Morgenstern G, Clink HM, et al. The place of bone-marrow transplantation in acute myelogenous leukaemia. Lancet 1980; I: 1047-1050.

CHAPTER 3

Meningeal involvement in patients with acute nonlymphocytic leukaemia: incidence, management and predictive factors

A.W. Dekker*, A. Elderson**, K. Punt*, and J.J. Sixma*

Departments of Haematology* and Neurology**, University Hospital Utrecht, The Netherlands

SUMMARY

Between 1977 and 1983 symptomatic meningeal leukaemia was diagnosed in 9 out of a total number of 93 adult patients with acute nonlymphocytic leukaemia (10%). All cases occurred after complete remission had been achieved (46 patients), either as the only site of relapse (three patients), or together with a first bone marrow relapse (three patients) or after a bone marrow relapse (three patients). Extra medullary involvement at initial diagnosis was the only independent predictive factor ($p < 0.005$), the number of patients with initial hyperleucocytosis being too small (three) for evaluation. Remission of the meningeal leukaemia was obtained after treatment in four out of eight patients. The presence of meningeal leukaemia and the response to therapy had no influence on survival. The morbidity and therapy related toxicity were impressive however, making prophylactic treatment in patients at risk highly desirable. Some recommendations for a prophylactic treatment scheme are suggested.

INTRODUCTION

An increase of meningeal leukaemia was observed in acute lymphoblastic leukaemia after remission induction therapy and maintenance therapy had improved substantially, leading to longer survival. The lower incidence of meningeal leukaemia in acute nonlymphocytic leukaemia (ANLL), despite the improvement of the length of survival, and the low incidence in chronic leukaemia suggest that specific characteristics of leukaemic cells are major contributing factors in the development of meningeal leukaemia. The proportion of adult patients with ANLL suffering from meningeal leukaemia reported in the literature is quite variable. In some studies the occurrence of meningeal leukaemia was rare, less than two percent (1-3), while others reported incidences higher than twenty percent (4,5). This difference can be partly explained by the fact that meningeal leukaemia in patients with ANLL at initial diagnosis and at the time of complete remission is often completely asymptomatic and is only found if the cerebrospinal fluid is investigated routinely (4,6,7,8). An incidence of less than ten percent was found when patients with a previous bone marrow relapse were excluded (5,7,9,10).

Central nervous system (CNS) prophylaxis has not been recommended as a routine for patients with ANLL because the incidence of meningeal leukaemia is relatively low and because this measure has not prolonged systemic remission (11). Definition of a specific subgroup of patients with an increased risk of meningeal leukaemia may be of value, however, because symptomatic meningeal leukaemia makes the patient very ill and the subsequent CNS therapy entails many toxic symptoms. Recognition of a subgroup at risk may lead to the use of, less toxic, CNS prophylaxis. Predictive factors for meningeal leukaemia in ANLL have not been clearly identified (7,10). Some authors have found a higher incidence in acute myelomonocytic leukaemia (6) or in acute monoblastic leukaemia (12).

We have studied the clinical data of 9 adult patients with symptomatic meningeal leukaemia caused by ANLL and have analysed the possible prognostic factors with their implications for prophylactic measures.

PATIENTS AND METHODS

Ninety-three patients were treated between 1977 and 1982, eighty-nine patients were treated at our own department (13) and four in an affiliated hospital.The remission induction treatment consisted of doxorubicin 50 mg/m^2 intravenously on day 1, vincristine 1 mg/m^2 i.v. on day 2 and cytosine arabinoside 80 mg/m^2 i.v. every 12 hours on day 3 to 8 (14). Patients were classified according to the FAB system (15). Standard criteria for diagnosis, remission and relapse were used. The diagnosis meningeal leukaemia was made if leukaemic blasts were found in stained slides prepared from 1 ml cerebrospinal fluid (CSF) after sedimentation (16). CNS remission was defined as clearance of leukaemic cells from the CSF with improvement of the neurological symptoms. Eight patients with meningeal leukaemia were treated twice weekly with intrathecal cytosine arabinoside (50 mg/m^2) and/or methotrexate (15 mgr) diluted in normal saline without preservative. Six patients received in addition cranial irradiation with 24 Gy. After CNS remission was achieved intrathecal therapy was continued monthly for six months. The results, reported in this study are as of December 1, 1982.

Statistical analysis

Survival and remission duration curves were analysed by standard life tables. Initial clinical features as possible prognostic factors were compared by the chi-square test with Yates correction or by the two-sample test of Wilcoxon.

Multivariate analysis by stepwise logistic regression (BMDP Statistical Software, 1981 Edition, University of California Press) to assess the role and independence of prognostic factors on disease free survival or on the occurrence of meningeal leukaemia was performed in the group of 46 complete responders out of 93 patients treated similarly in every respect between 1977 and 1982. The following variables were analysed: sex, fever or infection at admission (present or absent), morphologic subtype (FAB M1, M2, M3, M4, M5), haemoglobin ($>$ or $\leqslant$ 6 mmol/l), white blood cell count ($>$ or $\leqslant$ 100×10^9/l), platelet count ($>$ or $\leqslant$ 20×10^9/l), number of cytotoxic courses (1 to 4) and extramedullary involvement (present or absent). Extra medullary involvement was defined as splenomegaly ($>$ 5 cm below the costal margin) with or without hepatomegaly and/or lymphadenopathy (lymph nodes with a diameter of more than 2 cm in more than two lymph node regions). Skin or testicular infiltration alone was not encountered in the complete remission group. The Cox regression model for life table data was used for multivariate analysis of the variables mentioned and their relationship with disease free survival.

RESULTS

The overall incidence of meningeal leukaemia in ANLL between 1977 and 1983 was 9 out of 93 patients (10%). These 9 cases occurred among 46 complete responders (20%). Symptomatic meningeal leukaemia was not observed at initial diagnosis or during remission induction treatment. The median interval between first diagnosis and meningeal leukaemia was 7 months (range 2-22 months).

Symptoms and signs in meningeal leukaemia (Table 1)

The most frequent findings observed were those caused by increased intracranial pressure such as severe headache and papilloedema. Meningism was infrequent. Only one patient had fever at the time of diagnosis, probably due to a simultaneous bone marrow relapse. In the phase preceding overt meningeal leukaemia, the patients often had vague and non-specific symptoms such as paresthesias and brachialgia. In all patients leukaemic cells were easily identified in the CSF after sedimentation. The median cell count in the CSF at diagnosis was 161×10^6/l (range 8-3000). An increase of the CSF protein concentration was always observed, median protein content was 1.22

Table 1. Symptoms and signs in 9 patients with meningeal involvement in acute nonlympocytic leukaemia

Headache	7
Papilloedema	5
Meningism	3
Cranial nerve palsy	2
Root pain	4
Paresthesias	3
Fever	1
CSF abnormalities*	9
CAT scan abnormal**	3

* Leukaemic cells in the cerebrospinal fluid.
** Computerised axial tomography showed parenchymal deposits in 3 out of 8 patients.

g/l (0.50-4.1). This value was related to the degree of pleocytosis. A computerised axial tomography was performed in 8 patients. Two patients had cerebral infiltration and one patient had cerebellar abnormalities.

Treatment response and toxicity

Eight patients were treated: 6 patients received intrathecal cytosine arabinoside and 2 patients methotrexate as first therapy. Four patients achieved a remission with a median duration of 5 months, 1 after cytosine arabinoside alone and 3 after a combination of cytosine arabinoside with methotrexate or cranial irradiation. The median survival time after meningeal leukaemia had become manifest was 8 months (range $3\text{-}9^{+}$) for the responders and 10.5 months (range 2-14) for the non-responders. In only one case could the cause of death be attributed to meningeal leukaemia: simultaneous bone marrow relapse was the most important cause of death in 6 patients.

Intrathecal therapy by lumbar punctures was well tolerated, only one episode of chemical meningitis was observed. In 3 out of 5 patients with an intraventricular shunt (17) transient side effects such as headache, fever, dysarthria and dizziness occurred for a few hours after intraventricular administration of cytotoxic drugs.

Severe neurological abnormalities developed in 3 patients after intrathecal therapy and cranial irradiation. One patient with an ascending myelopathy had been treated before with a total dose of 1300 mg cytosine arabinoside; in another patient a cerebellar syndrome developed after 1000 mg cytosine arabinoside and 75 mg methotrexate. Because both patients had a small number of leukaemic cells in the CSF at that time and autopsy was not performed, it was not clear whether the previous intrathecal therapy has been the most important contributing factor. In the third patient a partial lesion of the conus medullaris and cauda equina became manifest when she was in remission after therapy with 1100 mg cytosine arabinoside.

Predictive factors for meningeal leukaemia

All 93 adult patients described here, were treated with the same remission induction therapy and received the same supportive care. Forty-six patients (49%) achieved complete remission, the complete response rate was significantly higher in patients younger than 50 years (68%) than in older patients (28%). All patients were treated with the same maintenance regimen. Nine cases of meningeal leukaemia among these patients occurred (20%), 3 as an initial relapse, 3 simultaneously with a bone marrow relapse and 3 after a previous bone marrow relapse (Table 2). The influence of possible predictive factors for meningeal leukaemia in this group of 46 patients was analysed

Table 2. Site of first relapse in 46 patients with acute nonlymphocytic leukaemia

Bone marrow*	37
Central nervous system	3
Central nervous system with simultaneous bone marrow relapse	3
No relapse	3

* Three CNS leukaemia in second or third relapse.

Table 3. Clinical data at diagnosis in 46 patients with acute nonlymphocytic leukaemia with or without subsequent meningeal leukaemia

	With meningeal leukaemia	Without meningeal leukaemia
Number of patients	9	37
Age (yr)*	35 (15-55)	43 (18-79)
Sex (M/F)	6/3**	15/22**
Extramedullary involvement°	5***	5***
WBC count (× 10^9/l)*	49 (3-253)°°	10 (0.3-136)°°
Platelet count (× 10^9/l)*	34 (13-114)	44 (3-217)
FAB subclass M1-M3/M4-M5	5/4	19/18
Remission duration (months)*	7 (2-15)	9 (2-59)
Survival duration (months)*	23.5 (4-28)	20 (5-60)

* Median (range).
** Not significant, $\chi^2 = 1.08$.
*** $0.05 > p > 0.02$, $\chi^2 = 5.25$.
° For lymphadenopathy only, $0.02 > p > 0.01$, $\chi^2 = 6.58$.
°° $p < 0.05$, two-sample test of Wilcoxon.

(Table 3). Patients with meningeal leukaemia were relatively younger and had higher WBC counts at initial diagnosis ($p < 0.05$) and possessed more often extramedullary localizations ($p<0.05$) especially lymphadenopathy ($p < 0.02$). No association was found with pretreatment platelet count or FAB subclasses. Stepwise logistic regression identified only extramedullary involvement at initial diagnosis as important predictive factor for meningeal leukaemia ($p = 0.005$). Three out of 15 patients with hyperleucocytosis (WBC count $> 100 \times 10^9/l$) at admission achieved complete remission during which meningeal leukaemia occurred in 2 of them. This number was too small for further statistical analysis.

Using the Cox regression model for life table data, only the presence of extramedullary involvement had a significant (negative) outcome on the duration of systemic remission ($p = 0.01$).

DISCUSSION

Meningeal leukaemia has been reported with increasing frequency in ANLL as a consequence of a longer duration of remission.

In this study 9 cases of symptomatic meningeal leukaemia were observed in 46 complete responders out of a total number of 93 adult patients with ANLL, the incidence thus being 20 percent. The incidence of meningeal leukaemia was 13 percent when three cases with a prior bone marrow relapse were excluded. All cases occurred after complete remission had been achieved. Remission induction therapy consisted of a combination of doxorubicin, vincristine and cytosine arabinoside in conventional doses. Although cytosine arabinoside penetrates into the CSF, a therapeutic level is apparently not reached with these doses (18,19). A contributing factor to this relatively high incidence of meningeal leukaemia might be our cytotoxic regimen used at that time.

The pathogenesis of meningeal leukaemia is not well known. The incidence and extent of leukaemic infiltration decreases from the dura mater to arachnoid and brain parenchyma (20,21). The presence of perivascular infiltrates in the arachnoid (21,22) and of leukaemic infiltrates extending along blood vessels between bone marrow of the skull and dura mater (23) support the hypothesis that the usual route of spread is contiguous extension at the time of active haematologic disease (24). It requires time before symptomatic meningeal leukaemia occurs, the central nervous system being a sanctuary site with slowly proliferating leukaemic cells (25). The median time from complete remission to meningeal leukaemia in our study was 7 months.

Remission of meningeal leukaemia was only achieved in 4 out of 8 patients who were treated. The occurrence of meningeal leukaemia and the response to therapy had no influence on survival. Despite the lack of impact on survival and the presence of only one death attributable to meningeal leukaemia, the quality of life in patients with symptomatic disease was poor. Patients had severe complaints and in three patients subacute neurotoxicity occurred after therapy: a severe myelopathy (two cases) and encephalopathy (one case).

The occurrence of asymptomatic meningeal leukaemia was not investigated in our patients. The incidence of asymptomatic disease at the time of initial diagnosis or after achievement of complete remission is approximately 7% (4,8), although occasionally a higher incidence has been reported (6). Treatment of asymptomatic disease is easier with less toxicity (7). The same is true for CNS prophylaxis which is quite effective (11) and perhaps possible with only a few intrathecal injections (26). Other authors (2,27) are of the opinion that because of the low incidence of meningeal leukaemia, the short survival of most patients, and the failure of CNS prophylaxis to prolong systemic remission, preventive therapy should not be recommended as a routine for adult patients with ANLL. However, we feel that it may be of value to identify a subgroup with a higher risk for meningeal leukaemia. We encountered meningeal leukaemia more often in male patients, in younger patients, in patients with a higher WBC count or with extramedullary involvement at diagnosis. Of these factors only the WBC count and extramedullary involvement were significantly associated. Extramedullary involvement at initial diagnosis was the only independent factor predicting meningeal leukaemia ($p = 0.005$). The relationship between a high WBC count, extramedullary involvement and meningeal leukaemia is well established for ALL (7,28,29). Some other studies have suggested that these factors may also be important in ANLL (6,7,10).

Our study does not allow us to draw reliable conclusions about the predictive value of hyperleucocytosis because we had too few patients. The course in these patients is highly suggestive however: of 3 patients with hyperleucocytosis who achieved complete remission, 2 developed meningeal leukaemia. A complicating factor in patients with hyperleucocytosis is the high incidence of early death (13,30-33), reducing the number of evaluable patients.

In some studies (5,6,21) a higher incidence of meningeal leukaemia was found in monocytic or myelomonocytic leukaemia. In our study (Table 3) this morphological subtype was not a predictive factor confirming other recent studies (7,10,34).

Thrombocytopenia was not a predictive factor for meningeal leukaemia. This is thus not consistent with the hypothesis (28) that small haemorrhages in severe thrombocytopenic patients provide a possible route for leukaemic cells to enter the CNS from the blood.

It remains difficult to predict the precise risk of meningeal leukaemia for a single patient. Despite the fact that at the present time meningeal leukaemia does not shorten survival, we wish to advocate some prophylactic measures for preventing the suffering caused by symptomatic meningeal leukaemia or caused by the toxicity of intensive intrathecal chemotherapy. Based on our present study we advise a diagnostic lumbar puncture as soon as remission has been reached in all patients. Asymptomatic meningeal leukaemia can then be treated adequately and with minor toxicity with intrathecal cytosine arabinoside (7,8,35).Patients with extramedullary involvement and/or hyperleucocytosis at diagnosis should be treated prophylactically. Because extramedullary involvement was the only predictive factor for meningeal leukaemia ($p = 0.005$) as well as for a shorter overall remission duration ($p = 0.01$) consolidation treatment with high dose cytosine arabinoside should also be considered in these patients. High dose cytosine arabinoside may eradicate resistant or residual leukaemic cells by achieving higher tissue concentrations also in sanctuary sites as the CNS (19,36).

ACKNOWLEDGEMEMTS

The authors thank Dr. J.A.J. Faber, Institute of Mathematical Statistics, University of Utrecht for statistical assistance and Annemiek Beyer and Maeyken Hoeneveld for secretarial help.

REFERENCES

1. Clarkson BD, Dowling MD, Gee TS, Cunningham IB, Burchenal JH. Treatment of acute leukemia in adults. Cancer 1975; 36: 775-779.
2. Whittaker JA. Advances in the management of adult acute myelogenous leukaemia. Br Med J 1980; 281: 960-964.
3. Armitage JO, Burns CP, Dick FR, Aunan SB, Slymen DJ. Results of aggressive chemotherapy for acute nonlymphoblastic leukemia in adults. Cancer Treat Rep 1982; 66: 1917-1924.
4. Wiernik PH, Schimpff SC, Shiffer ChA, Lichtenfeld JL, Aisner J, O'Connell MJ, Fortner C. Randomized clinical comparison of daunorubicin (NSC-82151) alone with a combination of daunorubicin, cytosine arabinoside (NSC-63878), 6-thioguanine (NSC-752), and pyrimethamine (NSC-3061) for the treatment of acute nonlymphocytic leukemia. Cancer Treat Rep 1976; 60: 41-53.
5. Lister TA, Whitebouse JMA, Oliver RTD, Bell R, Johnson SAM, Wrigley PFM, Ford JM, Cullen MH, Gregory W, Paxton AM, Malpas JS. Chemotherapy and immunotherapy for acute myelogenous leukemia. Cancer 1980; 46: 2142-2148.
6. Meyer RJ, Ferreira PPC, Cuttner J, Greenberg ML, Goldberg J, Holland JF. Central nervous system involvement at presentation in acute granulocytic leukemia. Am J Med 1980; 68: 691-694.
7. Stewart DJ, Keating MJ, McCredie KB, Smith TL, Youness E, Murphy SG, Bodey GP, Freireich EJ. Natural history of central nervous system acute leukemia in adults. Cancer 1981; 47: 184-196.
8. Yates J, Glidewell O, Wiernik P, Cooper R, Steinberg D, Dosik H, Levy R, Hoagland C, Henry P, Gottlieb A, Cornell C, Berenberg J, Hutchison JL, Raich P, Nissen M, Ellison R, Frelick R, James GW, Falkson G, Silver RT, Haurani F, Green M,

Henderson E, Leone L, Holland JF. Cytosine arabinoside with daunorubicin or adriamycin for therapy of acute myelocytic leukemia: A CALGB study. Blood 1982; 60: 454-462.
9. Glucksberg H, Cheever MA, Farewell VT, Fefer A, Sale GE, Thomas ED. High-dose combination chemotherapy for acute nonlymphoblastic leukemia in adults. Cancer 1981; 48: 1073-1081.
10. Shoenfeld Y, Rothenberg M, Berliner S, Gallant LA, Garfinkel D, Shaklai M, Pinkhas J. Absence of predictive parameters for CNS involvement in adult non-lymphocytic leukaemia at time of diagnosis. Scand J Haematol 1982; 28: 335-340.
11. Gale RP, Foon KA, Cline MJ, Zighelboim J, and the UCLA acute leukemia study group. Intensive chemotherapy for acute myelogenous leukemia. Annals Intern Med 1981; 94: 753-757.
12. Tobelem G, Jacquillat C, Chastang C, Auclerc M-F, Lechevallier T, Weil M, Daniel M-T, Flandrin G, Harrouseau J-L, Schaison G, Boiron M, Bernard J. Acute monoblastic leukemia: a clinical and biologic study of 74 cases. Blood 1980; 55: 71-76.
13. Dekker AW, Sixma JJ, Punt K. The management of acute non-lymphocytic leukaemia in adults. Neth J Med 1982; 25: 297-302.
14. Mathé G, Pouillart P, De Vassal F, Delgrado M, Schwarzenberg L, Misset JL, Hayat M, Jasmin C, Belpomme D, Musset M. Remission induction in acute lymphoid and acute myeloid leukaemias. Lancet 1976; I: 1130-1131.
15. Bennett JM, Catovsky D, Daniel M-T, Flandrin G, Galton DAG, Gralnick HR, Sultan C. Proposals for the classification of the acute leukaemias. Br J Haematol 1976; 33: 451-458.
16. Bots GThAM, Went LN, Schaberg A. Results of a sedimentation technique for cytology of cerebrospinal fluid. Acta Cytol 1964; 8: 234-241.
17. Ommaya AK. Subcutaneous reservoir and pump for sterile access to ventricular cerebrospinal fluid. Lancet 1963; II: 983-984.
18. Ho DHW. Potential advances in the clinical use of arabinosyl cytosine. Cancer Treat Rep 1977; 61: 717-722.
19. Breithaupt H, Pralle H, Eckhardt T, von Hattingberg M, Schick J, Loffler H. Clinical results and pharmacokinetics of high-dose cytosine arabinoside (HD ARA-C). Cancer 1982; 50: 1248-1257.
20. Moore EW, Thomas LB, Shaw RK, Freireich EJ. The central nervous system in acute leukemia. Arch Intern Med 1960; 105: 451-468.
21. Thomas LB. Pathology of leukemia in the brain and meninges: postmortem studies of patients with acute leukemia and of mice given inoculations of L1210 leukemia. Cancer Res 1965; 25: 1555-1571.
22. Price RA, Johnson WW. The central nervous system in childhood leukemia: I. The arachnoid. Cancer 1973; 31: 520-533.
23. Azzarelli B, Roessmann U. Pathogenesis of central nervous system infiltration in acute leukemia. Arch Pathol Lab Med 1977; 101: 203-205.
24. Lokich J, Galbo C. Leptomeningeal lymphoma: perspectives on management. Cancer Treat Rev 1981; 8: 103-110.
25. Tsuchiya J, Moteki M, Shimano S, Shinonome S, Suda T, Omine M, Maekawa T. Proliferative kinetics of the leukemic cells in meningeal leukemia. Cancer 1978; 42: 1255-1262.
26. Keating MJ, Smith TL, McCredie KB, Bodey GP, Hersh EM, Gutterman JU, Gehan E, Freireich EJ. A four-year experience with anthracycline, cytosine arabinoside vincristine and prednisone combination with acute leukemia. Cancer 1981; 47: 2779-2788.
27. Foon KA, Gale RP. Controversies in the therapy of acute myelogenous leukemia. Am J Med 1982; 72: 963-979.

28. West RJ, Graham-Pole J, Hardisty RM, Pike MC. Factors in pathogenesis of central-nervous-system leukaemia. Br Med J 1972; 3: 311-314.
29. Pavlovsky S, Eppinger-Helft M, Muriel FS. Factors that influence the appearance of central nervous system leukemia. Blood 1973; 42: 935-938.
30. Harris AL. Leukostasis associated with blood transfusion in acute myeloid leukaemia. Br Med J 1978; 1: 1169-1171.
31. Reiffers J, Raynal F, Broustet A. Acute myeloblastic leukemia in elderly patients. Treatment and prognostic factors. Cancer 1980; 45: 2816-2820.
32. Vaughan WP, Kimball AW, Karp JE, Dragon LH, Burke PhJ. Factors affecting survival of patients with acute myelocytic leukemia presenting with high Wbc counts. Cancer Treat Rep 1981; 65: 1007-1013.
33. Bell R, Rohatiner AZS, Slevin ML, Ford JM, Dhaliwal HS, Henry G, Birkhead RG, Amess JAL, Malpas JS, Lister TA. Short-term treatment of acute myelogenous leukaemia. Br Med J 1982; 284: 1221-1224.
34. Gordon S, Raik E, Hewitt B, Moore P. Cerebrospinal fluid involvement in patients with adult acute leukaemia and non-hodgkin's lymphoma. Austr/New Zeal J Med 1980; 10: 509-512.
35. Przuntek H, Breithaupt H. Cytarabine: Distribution in ventricular cerebrospinal fluid after lumbar injection. J Neurol 1981; 226: 3-76.
36. Pommier Y, Pochat L, Marie J-P, Zittoun RA. High-dose cytarabine in acute leukemia: toxicity and pharmacokinetics. Cancer Treat Rep 1983; 67: 371-373.

CHAPTER 4

Infection prevention during remission induction therapy

General considerations

INTRODUCTION

Infection is the most common cause of death during remission induction treatment in patients with acute nonlymphocytic leukaemia (ANLL) (1,2,3). Between 47 and 79 percent of causes of deaths among these patients are directly related to infectious episodes (4). Major predisposing factors are profound granulocytopenia, mucosal damage and acquisition of new microorganisms from the hospital environment (5).

There is an inverse correlation between the granulocyte count and both the incidence and severity of infection and febrile episodes (2,6,7). Because patients who are granulocytopenic have an impaired inflammatory response to the development of new infections, a minor infection in these patients may become life-threatening.

Also, as a consequence of cytotoxic agents there is some degree of mucosal damage along the alimentary canal and in the tracheobronchial tree. This may lead to infection with rapid progression, often with invasion of the blood stream by microorganisms.

The causative microorganisms are usually those which have already colonized the patient's alimentary canal, upper airways and/or skin. The most common organisms are aerobic gram-negative bacilli such as *Escherichia coli*, *Pseudomonas aeruginosa* and *Klebsiella pneumoniae* or gram-positive organisms (especially *Staphylococcus aureus*) (2,5). As was shown by Schimpff et al. in 1972, more than 80 percent of the microorganisms causing infection belongs to the patient's own endogenous microbial flora. Although nearly 50 percent of these microorganisms were acquired while the patient was in the hospital (1). These organisms from the hospital environment are often more likely to be resistant to commonly used systemic antimicrobial drugs than the original endogenous microbial flora. Therefore, a rational approach for infection prevention is to try to suppress the potential pathogens already colonizing the patient and to reduce acquisition with new microorganisms (5,8).

PREVENTION AGAINST EXOGENOUS MICROBIAL FLORA

Major sources of microorganisms acquired by the patient are hands of personnel, food, water and to a lesser degree, ambient air (9,10). Perhaps the most important route of transmission of potential pathogens from patient to patient is by the hands of hospital personnel. Medical personnel, however, frequently neglect simple handwashing and physicians are among the worst offenders (11). Food and beverages low in microbial counts, control of water supplies, attention to proper house keeping procedures and to careful hand washing procedures are all valuable measures for protecting the patient against the acquisition of new pathogens.

Another technique to reduce the acquisition of new pathogens is the use of reverse isolation procedures. Simple protective isolation alone, requiring isolation of the patient in a single room and all persons who enter the room to wear a gown, cap, mask and gloves, appears not to benefit granulocytopenic patients (12). Also the results of complete reverse isolation using a laminar air flow room or an equivalent setting are not convincing (13,14). Furthermore, this approach has several serious drawbacks. The isolation equipment is expensive and requires provision for a sterile supply and food service, skilled nursing staff and other services. Other liabilities are prolonged physical isolation and psychological deprivation.

MICROBIAL SUPPRESSION

Since the alimentary tract has been recognized as an important reservoir of potential pathogens, total decontamination of the alimentary tract has been investigated as a tool to prevent infections. The basic method of microbial suppression is the use of nonabsorbable antibiotics such as gentamicin, vancomycin and nystatin, often in conjunction with topical antiseptics applied to skin and orificia (8). The results of the use of decontamination of the gastrointestinal tract alone are controversial (8,13,15). This procedure was only significantly effective in preventing infections in one study (16). A poor compliance usually due to the unpleasant taste of the oral nonabsorbable antibiotic regimens can be accompanied by a significant risk of both rebound overgrowth of potential pathogens and acquisition of resistant strains (especially to gentamicin) from the hospital environment (5,8).

The combination of oral nonabsorbable antibiotics with complete isolation has improved these results. A substantial reduction (about 50 percent) in the incidence of infections with this combined approach was obtained in a number of studies (13,15-19). However in other studies results were less convincing (14,20).

SELECTIVE MICROBIAL SUPPRESSION

In the light of these problems another approach was developed by van der Waaij and colleagues (21-24). They determined the number of bacteria feeded to animals needed for colonization of the gastrointestinal tract. When an oral dose of bacteria was given to germ-free mice, they found that only very few microorganisms were already able to colonize the intestines. Many more bacteria were needed to colonize the alimentary tract of conventional mice with a normal gut flora. Also mice treated with broad spectrum antibiotics were rapidly colonized by low doses of oral gram-negative microorganisms. The apparent resistance to colonization of the alimentary tract of conventional mice was coined colonization resistance. Colonization resistance of the alimentary tract is a complex mechanism in which host factors and anaerobic microflora cooperate in limiting the colonization by potentially pathogenic microorganisms. This resistance to colonization was found to reside, in an important part, in the anaerobic intestinal flora (21). The susceptibility to colonization of germ-free mice and antibiotic treated mice was then explained by the absence of anaerobic bacteria in these mice. When this concept is true, antibiotics should be used for infection prevention that only affect the aerobic potential pathogens but not the anaerobic part of the gut flora. Because, when the anaerobic bacteria are eliminated the possibility of colonization by multiresistant aerobic bacteria, present in abundance in most hospitals, would than be enhanced. This approach seems suitable for infection prevention during remission induction treatment. Moreover, infections caused by anaerobes are relatively rare in these patients (1,2,25). Antibiotics which can eliminate the pathogenic aerobic gram-negative rods or yeasts from the gut without affecting the anaerobes are trimethoprim-sulfamethoxazole, nalidixic acid, neomycin, polymyxin (colistin), nystatin and amphotericin B (26). These drugs are more palatable leading to better compliance and also cheaper than gentamicin and vancomycin. Another advantage might be that because of the preservation of colonization resistance isolation procedures are less needed.

Alternative names used for selective microbial suppression are: selective decontamination, selective elimination, partial antibiotic decontamination, selective antimicrobial prophylaxis and selective antimicrobial modulation.

The results of clinical studies with trimethoprim- sulfamethoxazole alone, colistin plus trimethoprim- sulfamethoxazole and colistin plus neomycin used for selective decontamination are described in the next three chapters.

REFERENCES

1. Schimpff SC, Young VM, Greene WH, Vermeulen GD, Moody MR, Wiernik PH. Origin of infection in acute nonlymphocytic leukemia. Significance of hospital acquisition of potential pathogens. Ann Intern Med 77: 707-714, 1972.
2. Bodey GP, Rodriguez V, Chang H-Y, Narboni G. Fever and infection in leukemic patients. A study of 494 consecutive patients. Cancer 41: 1610-1622, 1978.
3. McCredie KB, Gehan EA, Freireich EJ, Mewlett JS, Coltman CA, Hussein KK, Balcerzak SP, Chen TT. Management of adult acute leukemia. A southwest oncology group study. Cancer 52: 958-966, 1983.
4. Young LS. Antimicrobial prophylaxis against infection in neutropenic patients. J Infect Dis 147: 611-614, 1983.
5. Pizzo PA, Schimpff SC. Strategies for the prevention of infection in the myelosuppressed or immunosuppressed cancer patient. Cancer Treat Rep 67: 223-234, 1983.
6. Bodey GP, Buckley M, Sathe YS, Freireich EJ. Quantitative relationships between circulating leukocytes and infection in patients with acute leukemia. Ann Intern Med 64: 328-340, 1966.
7. Gurwith MJ, Brunton JL, Lank BA, Ronald AR, Harding GKM. Granulocytopenia in hospitalized patients. I. Prognostic factors and etiology of fever. Am J Med 64: 121-126, 1978.
8. Schimpff SC. Infection prevention during profound granulocytopenia. New approaches to alimentary canal microbial suppression. Ann Intern Med 93: 358-361, 1980.
9. Remmington JS, Schimpff SC. Occasial notes. Please don't eat the salads. New Engl J Med 304: 433-435, 1981.
10. Pizzo PA. The value of protective isolation in preventing nosocomial infections in high risk patients. Am J Med 70: 631-637, 1981.
11. Albert RK, Condie F. Hand-washing patterns in medical intensive-care units. New Engl J Med 304: 1465-1466, 1981.
12. Nauseef WM, Maki DG. A study of the value of simple protective isolation in patients with granulocytopenia. New Engl J Med 304: 448-453, 1981.
13. Yates JW, Holland JF. A controlled study of isolation and endogenous microbial suppression in acute myelocytic leukemia patients. Cancer 32: 1490-1498, 1973.
14. Dietrich M, Gaus W, Vossen J, van der Waaij D, Wendt F. Protective isolation and antimicrobial decontamination in patients with high susceptibility to infection. A prospective cooperative study of gnotobiotic care in acute leukemia patients. I. Clinical results. Infection 5: 107-114, 1977.
15. Levine AS, Siegel SE, Schreiber AD, Hauser J, Preisler H, Goldstein IM, Seidler F, Simon R, Perry S. Bennett JE, Henderson ES. Protected environments and prophylactic antibiotics. A prospective controlled study of their utility in the therapy of acute leukemia. New Engl J Med 288: 477-483, 1973.
16. Schimpff SC, Greene WH, Young VM, Fortner CL, Jepsen L, Cusack N, Block JB, Wiernik PH. Infection prevention in acute nonlymphocytic leukemia. Laminar air flow room reverse isolation with oral, nonabsorbable antibiotic prophylaxis. Ann Intern Med 82: 351-358, 1975.
17. Rodriguez V, Bodey GP, Freireich EJ, McCredie KB, Gutterman JU, Keating MJ, Smith TL, Gehan EA. Randomized trial of protected environment – Prophylactic antibiotics in 145 adults with acute leukemia. Medicine 57: 253-266, 1978.
18. Buckner CD, Clift RA, Sanders JE, Meyers JD, Counts GW, Farewell VT, Thomas ED, and the Seattle marrow transplant team. Protective environment for marrow transplant recipients. A prospective study. Ann Intern Med 89: 893-901, 1978.

19. Bodey GP, McCredie KB, Keating MJ, Freireich EJ. Treatment of acute leukemia in protected environment units. Cancer 44: 431-436, 1979.
20. Lohner D, Debusscher L, Prevost JM, Klastersky J. Comparative randomized study of protected environment plus oral antibiotics versus oral antibiotics alone in neutropenic patients. Cancer Treat Rep 63: 363-368, 1979.
21. Van der Waaij D, Berghuis-de Vries JM, Lekkerkerk-van der Wees JEC. Colonization resistance of the digestive tract in conventional and antibiotic-treated mice. J Hyg (Camb) 69: 405-411, 1971.
22. Van der Waaij D, Berghuis JM, Lekkerkerk JEC. Colonization resistance of the digestive tract of mice during systemic antibiotic treatment. J Hyg (Camb) 70: 605-610, 1972.
23. Van der Waaij D, Berghuis-de Vries JM. Selective elimination of Enterobacteriaceae species from the digestive tract in mice and monkeys. J Hyg (Camb) 72: 205-211, 1974.
24. Van der Waaij D, Berghuis JM. Determination of the colonization resistance of the digestive tract of individual mice. J Hyg (Camb) 72: 379-387, 1974.
25. Pizzo PA, Robichaud KJ, Wesley R, Commers JR. Fever in the pediatric and young adult patient with cancer. A prospective study of 1001 episodes. Medicine 61: 153-165, 1982.
26. Van der Waaij D. Colonization resistance of the digestive tract as a major lead in the selection of antibiotics for therapy. In: Van der Waaij D, Verhoef J, eds. New criteria for antimicrobial therapy: maintenance of digestive tract colonization resistance. Amsterdam, Excerpta Medica: 271-282, 1979.

CHAPTER 5

Prevention of infection by trimethoprim-sulfamethoxazole plus amphotericin B in patients with acute nonlymphocytic leukaemia

Adriaan W. Dekker*, M.D., Maja Rozenberg-Arska**, M.D., Jan J. Sixma*,M.D. and Jan Verhoef**, M.D.

Departments of Haematology* and Clinical Bacteriology**, University Hospital Utrecht, The Netherlands

SUMMARY

Fifty-two patients with acute nonlymphocytic leukaemia were studied during remission induction treatment in a randomized trial to ascertain the effect of prophylactic oral trimethoprim-sulfamethoxazole on infection and fever rate. A decrease in the total number of acquired infections was found (16 infections in the group given trimethoprim-sulfamethoxazole versus 31 in the control group, $p < 0.01$). The number of patients without any infection in the trimethoprim- sulfamethoxazole group was 13 compared to only three in the control group ($p < 0.01$). Patients in the trimethoprim-sulfamethoxazole group needed parenteral antibiotics during 33% of the days they were granulocytopenic compared to 61% of these days for patients in the control group. However, six of nine bacteriologically documented infections in the trimethoprim-sulfamethoxazole group were caused by resistant microorganisms compared to two out of 20 in the control group.

INTRODUCTION

Infections are a frequent consequence of the severe granulocytopenia in patients with acute leukaemia (1). Patients with acute nonlymphocytic leukaemia are especially susceptible to bacterial infections during remission induction treatment. They usually become infected by aerobic gram-negative rods from the alimentary tract (2,3). The commonest infections are pneumonia, oesophagitis, pharyngitis, skin infections, and perianal and perirectal lesions. Various methods to prevent infections in these patients have been studied. The results of using protective isolation or prophylactic nonabsorbable antibiotics to prevent infection are not always convincing and comparable (4-6). Combinations of oral nonabsorbable antibiotics used for alimentary tract decontamination are often poorly tolerated, expensive, and do not always protect against acquisition of resistant microorganisms. Another approach has been suggested by van der Waay and coworkers (7,8): the selective suppression of the microbial flora in the gut. These workers have tried only to eliminate the aerobic flora of the alimentary tract. With the anaerobic flora left intact, the resistance to colonization by aerobic gram-negative rods is considered to be maintained and subsequent infection prevented. Antimicrobial agents such as trimethoprim-sulfamethoxazole, nalidixic acid, and colistin suppress only the aerobic flora. Therefore, these agents can be used for selective decontamination of the alimentary tract. The results of infection prevention by selective decontamination that have been evaluated are encouraging (9-11). Wade and colleagues (12) showed that the effect of the combination of trimethoprim-sulfamethoxazole and nystatin was comparable to that of the combination of gentamicin and nystatin. In another study (13) an additional benefit of using trimethoprim-sulfamethoxazole was reported on patients already receiving the combination of framycetin, colistin, and nystatin. However, all authors have concluded that more studies are needed before trimethoprim-sulfamethoxazole is used universally as a prophylactic antimicrobial in granulocytopenic patients.

We investigated the effect of prophylactically administered trimethoprim-sulfamethoxazole on the infection and fever rate in patients with acute nonlymphocytic leukaemia during remission induction treatment. We also investigated the influence of trimethoprim-sulfamethoxazole on the reduction of the need for systemically administered broad-spectrum antibiotics and on the emergence of resistant strains in these patients. We studied only patients with acute nonlymphocytic leukaemia because this group of patients is at the highest risk of developing infection due to the very low granulocyte counts in association with mucosal damage secondary to chemotherapy and because in the studies mentioned above only small numbers of these patients were evaluated.

PATIENTS AND METHODS

All adult patients with acute nonlymphocytic leukaemia, first diagnosed or in relapse, who were admitted to our hospital between 1 December 1978 and 1 November 1980 were randomized to a control group or to a group receiving trimethoprim-sulfamethoxazole prophylactically. Patients with fever and signs of infection at time of admission were also included but separately randomized. Patients who either did not qualify for remission induction treatment, or were allergic to trimethoprim-sulfamethoxazole or had signs of hepatic or renal failure were excluded. Trimethoprim- sulfamethoxazole (240 mg trimethoprim and 1200 mg sulfamethoxazole) was given orally twice daily, and amphotericin B (800 mg/d) was added to prevent colonization of the alimentary tract with yeasts; in both groups topical nystatin, 0.5×10^6 U every 4 hours, was used. No other prophylactic measures were taken. Patients were cared for in single rooms or in an open ward. The groups were similarly treated in every other respect. The antileukaemic treatment consisted of a combination of doxorubicin, cytarabine, and vincristine (14); sometimes thioguanine was added (15). The prophylactic treatment was started shortly before cytotoxic treatment was initiated and ended when the granulocyte count was above 500/µl and no further cytotoxic treatment was indicated.

Clinical investigations

Patients were daily examined for mucositis, cellulitis, or perianal lesions. Fever was defined as an oral temperature above 38°C lasting more than 12 hours. Clinically documented infections were defined as the presence of signs and symptoms of an infection not followed by a positive culture result. Bacteriologically documented infections were clinically documented infections in which pathogenic microorganism(s) could be isolated from the site of infection or from the blood. All granulocytopenic patients with suspected infections, fever or both were treated intravenously with gentamicin and cephalothin while the prophylactic treatment was continued.

Microbiological investigations

Surveillance cultures were obtained from the throat, nose, urine, and faeces of each patient at time of admission and thereafter once or twice weekly. Faecal samples were placed in transport medium containing cysteine-hydrochloride (Fluke; Aktien Gesellschaft, Buchs, Switzerland), peptone (Oxoid Ltd, Basingstoke, England), and yeast extract (Merck, Aktien Gesellschaft, Darmstadt, West Germany). After homogenization, 10-fold serial dilutions were made. For the isolation and enumeration of aerobic bacteria the dilutions were subcultured on MacConkey agar (Oxoid Ltd.), selective for gram-negative rods; blood agar (Blood Agar Base, with 7% defibrinated sheep blood, Oxoid Ltd.) for staphylococci and streptococci; and Sabouraud dextrose agar (Difco Laboratories, Detroit, Michigan), selective for yeasts. For the isolation and enumeration of anaerobic microorganisms serial dilutions were plated on blood agar containing Iso- sensitest agar (Oxoid Ltd.), 7% defibrinated sheep blood, 5% saponin (Merck), and kanamycin (125 µg/ml). For the first 20 patients, quantitative anaerobic samplings of stool were done. *Enterobacteriaceae* were identified with API 20 E (API System; S.A. La Balme, Les Grottes, France), anaerobic microorganisms with API 20A, and *Staphylococcus aureus* by deoxyribonuclease and coagulase assays. Antimicrobial susceptibility was tested by agar diffusion method on Isosensitest agar (Oxoid Ltd.) with Neo-sensitabs (Rosco; Taastrup, Denmark).

RESULTS

Fifty-eight patients were randomized, and 52 were evaluated (26 patients in each group). Of the six patients excluded from this study four died in the first days of induction therapy, one refused further therapy, and one patient developed allergic reactions to trimethoprim-sulfamethoxazole. Patients with infection at time of admission (eight in each group) were separately analyzed. The groups of patients were comparable in age, number of patients with first diagnosis or in relapse, number of anti-leukaemic courses, and response to therapy (Table 1).

Fever during granulocytopenia

As expected the prevalence of fever was high on days when patients were granulocytopenic, especially when the granulocyte count was lower than 100/µl; 30% of these days were associated with fever versus 46% in the control group ($p < 0.01$)(Table 2). The reduction in the number of days with fever and infection resulted in decreased use of intravenous antibiotics. Parenteral antibiotics were used 33% of the days patients were granulocytopenic in the trimethoprim-sulfamethoxazole group compared to 61% in the

Table 1. Clinical data from patients with acute nonlymphocytic leukaemia

	Control group	Trimethoprim-sulfamethoxazole
Patients, n	26	26
Age (mean), yrs	52	47
Patients infected at admission, n	8	8
First induction remission treatment, n	15	16
Antileukaemic courses (mean), n	1.5	1.8
Complete remissions, n	15	15
Partial remissions, n	2	3
Deaths during induction treatment, n	8	7
From infection	3	2
From haemorrhage	2	3
From infection + haemorrhage	2	2
From other cause	1	0
Thrombocytopenia* (mean ± SD), d	29 ± 12**	34.8 ± 16.9**
Granulocyte levels 101 to 499/µl (mean), d	10.4	10.5
Granulocyte levels < 100/µl (mean ± SD), d	17.9 ± 11.3°	27.8 ± 12.5°

* Thrombocyte levels < 100.000/µl.
** $p < 0.10$, unpaired t-test.
° $p < 0.01$, unpaired t-test.

Table 2. Fever and acquired infections in patients with acute nonlymphocytic leukaemia

	Control group	Trimethoprim-sulfamethoxazole
Patients, n	26	26
Fever and granulocyte levels		
Granulocyte levels 101 tot 499/µl, d	270	274
Associated with fever, d (%)	57* (21)	35* (13)
Granulocyte levels < 100/µl, d	458	725
Associated with fever, d (%)	209** (46)	215** (30)
Granulocyte levels > 500/µl, d	254	243
Associated with fever, d (%)	32 (13)	35 (14)
Patients without fever, n	0	5
Acquired infections, n	31***	16***
Bacteriologically documented infections	20°	9°
Major infections with bacteraemia	7	4
Major infections without bacteraemia	6	2
Minor infections	7	3
Clinically documented infections	11	7
Patients without acquired infections	3	13
Parenteral antibiotics during granulocytopenic°° periods (% of days)		
Including all patients	61	33
Excluding patients infected at admission	50	18

* $p > 0.05$ tested with the two-sample test of Wilcoxon.
** $p < 0.01$ tested with the two-sample test of Wilcoxon.
*** $p < 0.01$, $\chi^2 = 9.02$.
° $p < 0.05$, $\chi^2 = 5.80$.
°° Granulocytes < 500/µl.

control group. When patients with an infection at admission were excluded, this difference was more evident (Table 2).

Infections

A significant decrease ($p < 0.01$, $\chi^2 = 9.02$) in the number of acquired infections was found in the trimethoprim-sulfamethoxazole group (Table 2). There were 16 acquired infections (nine bacteriologically established, four of them with associated bacteraemias and seven clinically documented) compared to 31 in the control group (20 bacteriologically established, seven of them with associated bacteraemias and 11 clinically documented). Thirteen patients in the trimethoprim- sulfamethoxazole group had no infections compared to three in the control group ($p < 0.01$).

There was no difference in the frequency of bacteriologically documented pulmonary infections and septicaemias between the two groups. However, anorectal lesions, urinary tract infections, and skin lesions were less frequent in the trimethoprim-sulfamethoxazole group (Table 3).

Most of the bacteriologically confirmed infections were caused by gram-negative bacilli (Table 4). In the control group 13 of 20 and in the trimethoprim- sulfamethoxazole group seven of nine bacteriologically documented infections were caused by gram-negative rods ($\chi^2 = 2.93$, $0.05 < p < 0.10$). Most of these infections occurred on the days granulocyte counts were lower than 100/µl, in the control group 11 of 13 and in the trimethoprim-sulfamethoxazole group six of seven. Also, most of the infections caused by gram-positive microorganisms were present on these days.

The patients with infection at time of admission who at the same time were treated with parenteral antibiotics (eight in each group) were separately analyzed. In the group of patients with infection at admission who were receiving trimethoprim- sulfamethoxazole prophylactically, five infections were acquired, all caused by gram-negative rods. The total number of acquired infections in the control group was nine, and five were caused by gram-negative rods.

Amphotericin B prevented colonization of the lower alimentary tract with yeasts in the trimethoprim- sulfamethoxazole group. The prevalence of local extensive infections caused by *Candida* was two versus five in the control group. No disseminated candida infections were observed.

Microbiological surveillance

In patients receiving trimethoprim-sulfamethoxazole a reduction in the aerobic faecal gram-negative bacilli from 10^8 to 10^9 to less than 10^3 colony-forming units per gram of faeces was achieved in about 7 to 10 days. No influence of trimethoprim-sulfamethoxazole on the anaerobic faecal flora

Table 3. Sites of bacteriologically documented infections*

Infection	Control group	Trimethoprim-sulfamethoxazole
Pneumonia	3 (1)	2 (1)
Upper respiratory tract	0	1
Anorectal	4 (1)	1
Urinary tract	3 (1)	0
Skin and soft tissue	6	2
No site found ('septicaemia')	4 (4)	3 (3)
Total	20 (7)	9 (4)

* Parentheses indicate number of cases with bacteraemia.

Table 4. Microbiological documentation of infections and the prevalence of trimethoprim-sulfamethoxazole-resistant gram-negative bacilli*

	Control group		Trimethoprim-sulfamethoxazole	
Bacteriologically documented infections	20	(7)	9	(4)
Gram-positive bacteria	7	(3)	2	(1)
Staphylococcus aureus	4		1	
Streptococcus viridans	2	(2)	0	
Propionibacterium	1	(1)	0	
Eubacterium	0		1	(1)
Gram-negative bacteria	13**	(4)	7**	(3)
Escherichia coli	6	(2)	1	(1)
Klebsiella	2	(1)	1	(1)
Enterobacter	0		3	(1)
Serratia	1		0	
Pseudomonas aeruginosa	1		2	
E. coli + *Ps. aeruginosa*	3	(1)	0	
Acquisition and infection with trimethoprim-sulfamethoxazole-resistant gram-negative bacilli				
Transient° microorganisms	12		29	
Colonizing°° microorganisms	6	[2]	20	[6]
Escherichia coli	4	[2]	12	[1]
Klebsiella	1		2	[1]
Enterobacter	1		5	[3]
Pseudomonas aeruginosa	0		1	[1]

* Parentheses indicate number of cases with bacteraemia; brackets indicate number of cases with an infection.
** $p < 0.10$, $\chi^2 = 2.92$.
° Microorganisms appearing in one single culture. No cases with infection were seen.
°° Microorganisms appearing in consecutive cultures.

was seen (data not shown). In the control group, infections caused by *Escherichia coli* were predominant, whereas in the trimethoprim-sulfamethoxazole group *Enterobacter* species were the main causative agents. One of the main problems in using antibiotics prophylactically is the possible emergence of resistant microorganisms; therefore the emergence of gram-negative bacilli resistant to trimethoprim-sulfamethoxazole and infections caused by these microoorganisms was monitored (Table 4).

A distinction was made between resistant bacteria isolated only from a single surveillance culture (transient microorganisms), resistant bacteria that colonized the alimentary tract and that could be recovered from consecutive surveillance cultures, and resistant bacteria that caused subsequent infection. In the control group 12 patients acquired 18 strains of bacteria resistant to trimethoprim-sulfamethoxazole. Six of these strains colonized the alimentary tract, and two caused an infection, one of which was fatal. Some of the patients who harboured resistant microorganisms had been treated therapeutically with trimethoprim- sulfamethoxazole. In the group of patients given prophylactic trimethoprim-sulfamethoxazole, 19 patients acquired 49 resistant strains. Twenty of these strains colonized 14 patients, and six of the colonizing strains caused an infection, two of which were fatal. In both groups transient microorganisms did not cause any infection. Because the emergence of resistant gram-negative rods in both groups may have been caused by the use of parenteral antibiotics, we studied the influence of parenteral antibiotics on the emergence of resistant gram-negative rods. A high prevalence of colonization and subsequent infection with resistant strains was seen among the patients who had an infection at admission, especially those receiving trimethoprim-sulfamethoxazole prophylactically (13 resistant strains colonized seven patients; four of them led to infections) compared to the control group (two resistant strains colonized two patients without any infection). In the group of patients not infected at admission and receiving the prophylactic regimen, five of 10 patients who were treated at some point with parenteral antibiotics were colonized by resistant strains with two subsequent infections. Thirteen patients were not treated with parenteral antibiotics; in this group, two colonizations (without subsequent infection) by trimethoprim-sulfamethoxazole-resistant strains occurred.

Death rate and side effects

The death rate in both groups was about the same, and no difference in causes of death was found (Table 1). Trimethoprim-sulfamethoxazole was well tolerated; only one patient had to be excluded because of an allergic reaction. There was only a slight difference in the mean duration of thrombocytopenia ($0.10 > p > 0.05$) (Table 1). However, a significant increase of the mean duration of granulocytopenia in the trimethoprim- sulfamethoxazole group was found. The mean number of days with granulocyt counts lower than 100/µl was 17.9 ± 11.3 in the control group and 27.8 ± 12.5 in the trimethoprim-sulfamethoxazole group ($p < 0.01$). No difference between the two groups was seen in days with granulocyte counts at 101 to 499/µl and more than 500 granulocytes/µl.

DISCUSSION

In this randomized trial we evaluated the efficacy of the prophylactic administration of trimethoprim- sulfamethoxazole on the rate of infections during remission induction treatment in patients with acute nonlymphocytic leukaemia. Trimethoprim-sulfamethoxazole was chosen because it selectively suppresses the aerobic microbial flora in the gut and does not affect the anaerobic flora; therefore it could potentially preserve the colonization resistance (7,8). Moreover, trimethoprim-sulfamethoxazole is generally well tolerated and relatively inexpensive. All patients were cared for in single rooms or in conventional wards. They received nonsterile food. The administration of trimethoprim-sulfamethoxazole together with amphotericin B to patients in one of the groups was the only difference between the groups. Amphotericin B was added to the trimethoprim-sulfamethoxazole regimen because in a previous study by Hughes and associates (16) a higher prevalence of candida infections was seen in patients receiving high doses of trimethoprim- sulfamethoxazole.

A significant reduction in the number of acquired infections was shown in the group of patients with trimethoprim-sulfamethoxazole (31 episodes of infections in the control group compared to 16 infections in the trimethoprim-sulfamethoxazole group). The prevalence especially of anorectal, urinary tract, and skin or soft tissue infections was reduced, but no significant reduction in the frequency of pneumonias and bacteraemias was seen. Consequently, the need for intravenous antibiotics was significantly decreased. That the control group did not receive amphotericin B might have been a disadvantage. However, the addition of amphotericin B to the trimethoprim-sulfamethoxazole regimen is unlikely to have obscured the effect of trimethoprim-sulfamethoxazole, because the prevalence of bacterial infections especially was reduced in the group of patients receiving the prophylactic regimen. No influence of the amphotericin B, trimethoprim- sulfamethoxazole regimen was observed on the rate of colonization of the upper alimentary tract by yeasts (14 versus nine in the control group). The candida infections (two versus five in the control group) were all localized to the upper alimentary tract, and no disseminated candida infections were found in either group.

No increase in the number of infections caused by microorganisms intrinsically resistant to trimethoprim- sulfamethoxazole such as *Pseudomonas* or anaerobic microorganisms was seen. It was rather disturbing, however, that all infections caused by gram-negative microorganisms in patients of the trimethoprim- sulfamethoxazole group were caused by bacteria resistant to this drug. Despite the use of high doses of trimethoprim-sulfamethoxazole (480 mg and 2400 mg daily) a high frequency of colonization and subsequent infections by gram-negative bacilli resistant to this drug was found. Our findings are in contrast with those of previous reports that did not stress the occurrence of resistant microorganisms in patients receiving long-term trimethoprim-sulfamethoxazole (10-13,16). Most resistant strains were isolated from patients treated with trimethoprim-sulfamethoxazole and at the same time with parenteral broad-spectrum antibiotics such as cephalothin and gentamicin. But resistant bacteria also could be recovered from patients being treated with trimethoprim-sulfamethoxazole without parenteral antibiotics. This indicates that during the use of prophylactic trimethoprim-sulfamethoxazole the colonization resistance of the alimentary tract was not always maintained. Colonization and infection by resistant microorganisms occurred especially in patients who were infected at time of admission and who received both parenteral antibiotics and trimethoprim- sulfamethoxazole. This suggests that patients admitted with an infection have no benefit of selective decontamination with trimethoprim-sulfamethoxazole. Adding an oral nonabsorbable antimicrobial agent to the trimethoprim-sulfamethoxazole regimen might be advisable in periods when defects in the colonization resistance can be expected. We are, therefore, studying the effect of trimethoprim-sulfamethoxazole together with colistin on the prevention of colonization and infection by resistant microorganisms in patients with acute nonlymphocytic leukaemia. More studies are needed in human to evaluate the effect of antibiotics and cytotoxic drugs on the colonization resistance.

Nearly all infections (85%) occurred in patients with granulocyte counts lower that 100/µl, suggesting that prophylactic antibiotics should be given only to patients with profound and prolonged granulocytopenia.

Another potential disadvantage of the use of prophylactic trimethoprim-sulfamethoxazole could be the significantly increased duration of the granulocytopenic period. The mean duration of the granulocytopenic period in the control group was 28 days, comparable with that reported in other studies (11,13,17,18). However, in the trimethoprim-sulfamethoxazole group the mean length of this period was 38 days. The difference in the length of the thrombocytopenic periods between the groups was only marginal. Whether this finding should be attributed to a bone marrow-depressing effect of the large doses of trimethoprim-sulfamethoxazole used is not certain. Further studies are needed to answer this question.

Although our study showed that the use of trimethoprim-sulfamethoxazole reduced the prevalence of infections in patients with severe granulocytopenia, the large scale use of trimethoprim-sulfamethoxazole in those patients could have serious side effects. Therefore, before a decision on the routine use of trimethoprim-sulfamethoxazole in granulocytopenic patients is made, the potential disadvantages of such an approach must be weighed carefully. A regimen including colistin as a nonabsorbable antimicrobial together with amphotericin B and nystatin in addition to trimethoprim-sulfamethoxazole might be wiser. During the prophylactic treatment regular surveillance cultures are mandatory, especially when parenteral antibiotics are used.

ACKNOWLEDGEMENTS

The authors thank Prof.D. van der Waay, M.D., for his helpful advice and K. Punt, M.D., for critial reading of the manuscript; Mrs. G.A. Elsendoorn and Ms. M.A.T. Dekker for technical assistance; and Ms. Y. Joseph and Ms. A. Beijer for their patient secretarial assistance.

Grant support: in part by Hoffmann-La Roche, Basel, Switzerland.

REFERENCES

1. Bodey GP, Buckley M, Sathe YS, Freireich EJ. Quantitative relationships between circulating leukocytes and infection in patients with acute leukemia. Ann Intern Med 1966; 64: 328-340.
2. Schimpff SC, Young VM, Greene WH, Vermeulen GD, Moody MR, Wiernik PH. Origin of infection in acute nonlymphocytic leukemia: significance of hospital acquisition of potential pathogens. An Intern Med 1972; 77: 707-714.
3. Bodey GP, Rodriquez V, Chang H-Y, Narboni G. Fever and infection in leukemic patients: a study of 494 consecutive patients. Cancer 1978; 41: 1610-1622.
4. Schimpff SC. Infection prevention during profound granulocytopenia: new approaches to alimentary canal microbial suppression. Ann Intern Med 1980; 93: 358-361.
5. Infection prevention in acute leukaemia. Lancet 1978; 2: 769-770. Editorial.
6. Dietrich M, Gaus W, Vossen J. van der Waay D. Protective isolation and antimicrobial decontamination in patients with high susceptibility to infection. Infection 1977; 2: 107-114.
7. Van der Waay D, Berghuis JM, Lekkerkerk JEC. Colonization resistance of the digestive tract of mice during systemic antibiotic treatment. J Hyg (Camb) 1972; 70: 605-610.
8. Van der Waay D, Berghuis-De Vries JM. Selective elimination of Enterobacteriaceae species from the digestive tract in mice and monkeys. J Hyg (Camb) 1974; 72: 205-211.
9. Guiot HFL, van Furth R. Partial antibiotic decontamination. Br Med J 1977; 1: 800-802.
10. Sleijfer DT, Mulder NH, de Vries-Hospers HG, et al. Infection prevention in granulocytopenic patients by selective decontamination of digestive tract. Eur J Cancer 1980; 16: 859-869.
11. Gurwith MJ, Brunton JL, Lank BA, Harding GLM, Ronald AR. A prospective controlled investigation of prophylactic trimethoprim/sulfamethoxazole in hospitalized granulocytopenic patients. Am J Med 1979; 66: 248-256.
12. Wade JC, Schimpff SC, Hargadon MT, Fortner CL, Young VM, Wiernik PH. A comparison of trimethoprim- sulfamethoxazole plus nystatin with gentamicin plus nystatin in the prevention of infections in acute leukaemia. N Engl J Med 1981; 304: 1057-1062.
13. Enno A, Catovsky D, Darrell J, Goldman JM, Hows J, Galton DAG. Co-trimoxazole for prevention of infection in acute leukaemia. Lancet 1978; 2: 395-397.
14. Mathé G, Pouillart P, de Vassal F, et al. Remission induction in acute lymphoid and acute myeloid leukaemias. Lancet 1976; 1: 1130-1131.
15. Gale RP, Cline MJ. High remission-induction rate in acute myeloid leukaemia. Lancet 1977; 1: 497-499.

16. Hughes WT, Kuhn S, Chaudhary S, et al. Successful chemoprophylaxis for *Pneumocystis carinii* pneumonitis. N Engl J Med 1977; 297: 1419-1426.
17. Dekker AW, Rozenberg-Arska M, Verhoef J. Fever and infection in patients with acute non-lymphocytic leukaemia during induction treatment. In: Van der Waay D, Verhoef J, eds. New Criteria for Antimicrobial Therapy: Maintenance of Digestive Tract Colonization Resistance. Amsterdam: Excerpta Medica; 1979: 105-112.
18. Storring RA, Jameson B, McElwain TJ, Wiltshaw E, Spiers ASD, Gaya H. Oral non-absorbed antibiotics prevent infection in acute non-lymphoblastic leukaemia. Lancet 1977; 2: 837-840.

CHAPTER 6

Colistin and trimethoprim-sulfamethoxazole for the prevention of infection in patients with acute nonlymphocytic leukaemia. Decrease in the emergence of resistant bacteria

M. Rozenberg-Arska*, A.W. Dekker**, J. Verhoef*

Departments of Clinical Bacteriology* and Haematology**, University Hospital Utrecht, The Netherlands

SUMMARY

In a previous study we demonstrated that trimethoprim- sulfamethoxazole decreases the prevalence of infection in patients with severe granulocytopenia. However, treatment was accompanied by a relatively high incidence of multiresistant microorganisms. We therefore conducted this study to determine whether the addition of colistin to the trimethoprim- sulfamethoxazole regimen prevents the emergence of these resistant bacteria. Thirty consecutive adult patients with acute nonlymphocytic leukaemia received trimethoprim-sulfamethoxazole plus colistin p.o. prophylactically. The results of this study were compared with the results of our previously published controlled study. Trimethoprim-sulfamethoxazole plus colistin was as effective as trimethoprim- sulfamethoxazole in preventing infection. However, the addition of colistin significantly reduced the acquisition of and infection by gram-negative bacilli which were resistant to trimethoprim-sulfamethoxazole. Only two patients were colonized with resistant strains, and no infections with these strains were observed. We have concluded that patients with acute nonlymphocytic leukaemia should receive a combination of trimethoprim-sulfamethoxazole plus colistin prophylactically during remission induction treatment.

INTRODUCTION

Infections are still the major cause of morbidity and mortality during remission induction treatment in patients with acute nonlymphocytic leukaemia (1,2). Most of these infections are caused either by aerobic gram-negative bacilli normally found in the faecal flora, or by hospital-acquired microorganisms which colonize the alimentary tract during hospitalization (3-5). The incidence of acquired infections can be significantly reduced by administering antimicrobial drugs that selectively suppress the aerobic flora of the alimentary tract and at the same time preserve the anaerobic flora (6). Several recent studies have shown that prophylactic administration of oral trimethoprim- sulfamethoxazole reduces the incidence of acquired infections caused by *Enterobacteriaceae* in patients with severe granulocytopenia (7-9). We found a significant reduction in the total number of acquired infections in a group of patients who received trimethoprim-sulfamethoxazole prophylactically (9). However, we were disturbed by the fact that the acquisition rate of trimethoprim-sulfamethoxazole resistant *Enterobacteriaceae* was much higher in the group of patients receiving this drug; some of these strains caused serious infections. Colonization of the alimentary tract by resistant *Enterobacteriaceae* during treatment with trimethoprim-sulfamethoxazole has also been found in several other recent studies (10-15).

In the present study we attempted to reduce the emergence of resistant microorganisms by adding colistin to the trimethoprim-sulfamethoxazole regimen.

PATIENTS AND METHODS

Thirty-three consecutive adult patients with acute nonlymphocytic leukaemia, first diagnosed or in relapse, were admitted to our hospital between November 30, 1980 and December 1, 1981; they received oral antimicrobial prophylaxis to prevent infection during remission induction treatment. This prophylactic regimen consisted of trimethoprim-sulfamethoxazole (240 mg trimethoprim and 1200 mg sulfamethoxazole) administered every 12 h and colistin sulfate tablets (150 mg) administered every 6 h. The patients also received antifungal prophylaxis with amphotericin B tablets (800 mg/day). Whenever yeasts were found in surveillance cultures from the throat, a topical nystatin suspension (4 million units/day) was added. Patients were nursed in single rooms or in an open ward. The antileukaemic treatment was as previously described (9) and consisted of an anthracycline- cytarabine combination with vincristine; during relapse, thioguanine was also added.

The prophylactic regimen was started before the initiation of cytotoxic drugs and was continued until the granulocyte count exceeded 500/µl and no further cytotoxic treatment was indicated. Surveillance cultures from the nose, throat and urine as well as faeces samples were obtained at admission, and once or twice weekly thereafter. The microbiological methods used to isolate and identify bacteria were the same as described previously (9), except that anaerobic stool cultures were not done in this study.

All febrile granulocytopenic patients (oral temperature above 38°C for more than 12 h) were treated with a combination of gentamicin and cefuroxime. Antibiotic adjustments were made when indicated.

RESULTS

Thirty-three patients with acute nonlymphocytic leukaemia took part in the study, 30 of whom could be evaluated. The clinical data of these patients are shown in Table 1.

Fever was observed on 32% of the days during which the patients had severe granulocytopenia (less than 100 cells/µl). Parenteral antimicrobial agents were used on 37% of the days during which patients were suffering from granulocytopenia.

The group of patients receiving trimethoprim- sulfamethoxazole plus colistin was comparable (with respect to age, number of infections at admission, remission-relapse status and the duration of aplasia caused by the same cytotoxic regimens) to the patients in our previous study (9) who were treated with trimethoprim-sulfamethoxazole only. Therefore, we decided to compare the results from both groups (Tables 1 and 2).

Fourteen acquired infections were observed in the group of patients who received trimethoprim- sulfamethoxazole plus colistin as compared with 16 in the group who received trimethoprim-sulfamethoxazole only. Six infections could be documented microbiologically in the trimethoprim-sulfamethoxazole plus colistin group (Table 2). Only one patient suffered from an infection due to *Enterobacteriaceae*. In surveillance cultures from 12 patients, trimethoprim-sulfamethoxazole-resistant strains could be recovered

Table 1. Clinical data from patients with acute nonlymphocytic leukaemia

	Trimethoprim-sulfamethoxazole	Trimethoprim-sulfamethoxazole + colistin
Patients (n)	26	30
Mean age (yrs)	47	46
Patients infected at admission (n)	8	9
First induction remission treatment (n)	16	17
Antileukaemic courses (mean) (n)	1.8	1.8
Complete remissions (n)	15	15
Deaths during induction treatment (n)	7	7
caused by infection	2	2
caused by haemorrhage	3	4
caused by infection + haemorrhage	2	1
Granulocyte count 101 to 499/µl (mean) (d)	10.5	7.4
Granulocyte count < 100/µl (mean ± SD) (d)	27.8 ± 12.5	28.1 ± 16.1
associated with fever (%)	30	32
Parenteral antibiotics during granulocytopenic periods (% of days)	33	37

Table 2. Microbiological documentation of acquired infections and the prevalence of trimethoprim-sulfamethoxazole resistant gram-negative bacilli

	Trimethoprim-sulfamethoxazole		Trimethoprim-sulfamethoxazole + colistin	
Patients (n)	26		30	
Acquired infections (n)	16		14	
Bacteriologically documented infections*	9	(4)	6	(2)
aerobic gram-positive bacteria	1		1	
aerobic gram-negative bacteria	7	(3)	4	(1)
Enterobacteriaceae	5	(3)	1	
Pseudomonas	2		3	(1)
anaerobic bacteria	1	(1)	1	(1)
Clinically documented infections	7		8	
Patients without acquired infections	13		17	
Acquisition of and infection by trimethoprim-sulfamethoxazole resistant gram-negative bacilli				
Transient** microorganisms/patients	29/16		10/10	[1]
Colonizing° microorganisms/patients	20/14°°	[6]	2/2°°	[0]
Enterobacteriaceae	19	[5]	2	
Pseudomonas	1	[1]	-	

* Parentheses indicate number of cases with bacteraemia; brackets indicate number of cases with a subsequent infection.
** Microorganisms appearing in one single culture.
° Microorganisms appearing in consecutive cultures.
°° $p < 0.001$, $\chi^2 = 15.19$.

during prophylactic treatment with trimethoprim-sulfamethoxazole plus colistin. Colonization of the lower alimentary tract by resistant strains only occurred in two patients (compared with 14 patients in our previous group). Only one resistant *Enterobacteriaceae* strain caused an infection (compared with five infections in the trimethoprim-sulfamethoxazole group, three of which were associated with bacteraemias; see Table 2). No colistin-resistant strains could be recovered from the surveillance cultures. *Pseudomonas* infections (skin and soft tissue infections with one associated bacteraemia) occurred in three patients without any previous evidence of these bacteria in surveillance cultures (Table 2).

A rapid reduction in aerobic gram-negative rods in the faeces of patients receiving trimethoprim- sulfamethoxazole plus colistin was observed within four days; this was usually achieved after seven to ten days during treatment with trimethoprim-sulfamethoxazole alone (data not shown).

The combination of trimethoprim-sulfamethoxazole plus colistin was well tolerated. Two patients developed an allergic reaction (probably due to sulpha components) and were treated with trimethoprim (200 mg every 12 h) and colistin.

DISCUSSION

In a previous study (9) we observed a significant reduction in the number of acquired infections in patients with acute nonlymphocytic leukaemia who received trimethoprim-sulfamethoxazole during remission induction treatment. However, it was rather disturbing that all the infections caused by gram-negative microorganisms were due to trimethoprim- sulfamethoxazole resistant bacteria. To prevent the emergence of these resistant strains, we therefore decided to treat patients with acute nonlymphocytic leukaemia with a prophylactic regimen of trimethoprim- sulfamethoxazole plus colistin during remission induction treatment. With the exception of *Proteus spp.*, most aerobic gram-negative microorganisms are sensitive to colistin, which is not absorbed from the gastrointestinal tract. Because of the relatively high incidence of resistant microorganisms (9-15) in patients receiving only trimethoprim-sulfamethoxazole, we felt it would be rather hazardous in our hospital to study the efficacy of this combination in a controlled fashion, i.e. including a control group of patients receiving trimethoprim-sulfamethoxazole alone. However, from the clinical data of the 30 patients who received trimethoprim-sulfamethoxazole plus colistin, we concluded that this group of patients was comparable in all respects to the group of patients from our previous study (9). Therefore, we decided to include these data in Tables 1 and 2. The combination of trimethoprim- sulfamethoxazole plus colistin was well tolerated in our patients, and its efficacy in preventing infections was at least as good as trimethoprim-sulfamethoxazole alone. The addition of colistin significantly reduced the acquisition rate of and the number of infections by resistant *Enterobacteriaceae*.

On the basis of our results, we feel that patients with acute nonlymphocytic leukaemia who are undergoing remission induction treatment should be treated prophylactically with a combination of trimethoprim- sulfamethoxazole and colistin rather than with trimethoprim-sulfamethoxazole alone.

ACKNOWLEDGEMENT

The authors thank Miss. Y. Joseph for her secretarial assistance.

REFERENCES

1. Keating, M.J., Smith, T.L, McCredie, K.B., Bodey, G.P., Hersh, E.M., Gutterman, J.U., Gehan, E., Freireich, E.J.: A four-year experience with anthracycline, cytosine

arabinoside, vincristine and prednisone combination chemotherapy in 325 adults with acute leukemia. Cancer 47 (1981) 2779-2788.

2. Glucksberg, H., Cheever, M.A., Farewell, V.T., Fefer, A., Scale, G.E., Thomas, E.D.: High-dose combination chemotherapy for acute non-lymphoblastic leukaemia in adults. Cancer 48 (1981) 1073-1081.
3. LeFrock, J.L., Ellis, C.A., Weinstein, L.: The impact of hospitalization on the aerobic fecal microflora. Am. J. Med. Sci. 277 (1979) 269-274.
4. Newman, K.A., Schimpff, S.C., Young, M., Wiernik, P.H.: Lessons learned from surveillance cultures in patients with acute non-lymphocytic leukaemia. Usefulness for epidemiologic, preventive and therapeutic research. Am. J. Med. 70 (1981) 423-432.
5. Schimpff, S.C.: Surveillance cultures. J. Infect. Dis. 144 (1981) 81-84.
6. Waaij, D.van der, Berghuis-de Vries, J.M.: Selective elimination of *Enterobacteriaceae* species from the digestive tract in mice and monkeys. J. Hyg. (Camb.) 71 (1974) 205-211.
7. Gurwith, M.J., Brunton, J.L., Lank, B.A., Harding, G.L.M., Ronald, A.R.: A prospective controlled investigation of prophylactic trimethoprim- sulfamethoxazole in hospitalized granulocytopenic patients. Am. J. Med. 66 (1979) 248-256.
8. Wade, J.C., Schimpff, S.C., Hargadon, M.T., Fortner, C.L., Young, V.M., Wiernik, P.H.: A comparison of trimethoprim-sulfamethoxazole plus nystatin with gentamicin plus nystatin in the prevention of infections in acute leukaemia. N. Engl. J. Med. 304 (1981) 1057-1062.
9. Dekker, A.W., Rozenberg-Arska, M., Sixma, J.J., Verhoef, J.: Prevention of infection by trimethoprim-sulfamethoxazole plus amphotericin B in patients with acute non-lymphocytic leukaemia. Ann. Intern. Med. 95 (1981) 555-559.
10. Wilson, J.M., Guiney, D.G.: Failure of oral trimethoprim-sulfamethoxazole prophylaxis in acute leukaemia. Isolation of resistant plasmids from strains of *Enterobacteriaceae* causing bacteremia. N. Engl. J. Med. 306 (1982) 16-20.
11. Jacoby, G.A.: Editorial. Perils of prophylaxis. N. Engl. J. Med. 306 (1982) 43-44.
12. De Jongh, C.A., Schimpff, S.C., Wiernik, P.H.: (Letter): Antibiotic prophylaxis in acute leukemia. Ann. Intern. Med. 95 (1981) 783-784.
13. Young, L.S.: Editorial. Trimethoprim- sulfamethoxazole and bacterial infections during leukaemic therapy. Ann. Intern. Med. 95 (1981) 508-509.
14. Towner, K.J., Pearson, N.J., Pinn, P.A., O'Grady, F.: Increasing importance of plasmid mediated trimethoprim resistance in enterobacteria: two six-month clinical surveys. Br. Med. J. 280 (1980) 517-519.
15. Murray, B.E., Rensimer, E.R., DuPont, H.L.: Emergence of high level trimethoprim resistance in fecal *Escherichia coli* during oral administration of trimethoprim or trimethoprim- sulfamethoxazole. N. Eng. J. Med. 306 (1982) 130-135.

CHAPTER 7

The prevention of infections in acute leukaemia: a comparison of colistin plus neomycin with colistin plus trimethoprim-sulfamethoxazole

A.W. Dekker*, M. Rozenberg-Arska**, and J. Verhoef**

Departments of Haematology* and Clinical Bacteriology**, University Hospital Utrecht, The Netherlands

SUMMARY

In thirty patients with acute leukaemia infection prevention during remission induction treatment was studied in a randomized trial comparing nonabsorbable antibiotics, colistin plus neomycin (CN), with a combination of nonabsorbable and absorbable antibiotics, colistin plus trimethoprim-sulfamethoxazole (CT). Both regimens were similarly effective in preventing infections caused by aerobic gram-negative microorganisms (three infections in the CN group and two in the CT group). The addition of trimethoprim-sulfamethoxazole to colistin reduced the number of infections caused by gram-positive bacteria (one infection without bacteraemia in the CT group versus seven infections with four bacteraemias in the CN group, $p<0.05$). In only one patient belonging to the CT group colonization with subsequent infection, caused by resistant microorganisms, occurred. Four patients of the CT group developed allergic reactions, three of them continued with trimethoprim only. It can be concluded that both regimens are effective in the prevention of infections caused by aerobic gram-negative bacilli. The combination of colistin plus trimethoprim-sulfamethoxazole is preferable because the systemic activity of trimethoprim-sulfamethoxazole seems to decrease the occurrence of infections and septicaemias caused by gram-positive bacteria.

INTRODUCTION

Selective decontamination of the alimentary tract, with preservation of the colonization resistance, is at present the most promising approach for prevention of infections in patients with severe granulocytopenia (1-4). Several prospective randomized studies based on this principle have shown a significant reduction of infections caused by aerobic gram-negative bacilli (5-9). For selective decontamination both absorbable (trimethoprim-sulfamethoxazole, nalidixic acid) and nonabsorbable (polymyxin (colistin), neomycin or tobramycin, amphotericin B, nystatin) antimicrobial drugs can be used (10-12). It is not clear whether systemic antibiotic activity in addition to selective decontamination has any value. Absorbable antimicrobial agents may lead to toxic or allergic reactions. The E.O.R.T.C. Gnotobiotic Project Group (13) started a prospective randomized study to compare colistin plus neomycin (CN) with colistin plus trimethoprim-sulfamethoxazole (CT) to answer the following questions: (1) are both regimens useful for selective decontamination?, (2) does the systemic antibiotic activity of trimethoprim-sulfamethoxazole improve the clinical results of selective decontamination?, (3) is there a difference in the duration of the granulocytopenic period and in the incidence of allergic reactions between the two regimens? The results obtained with 30 patients from our department are described here. These preliminary data will be followed later by the results of the entire trial.

PATIENTS AND METHODS

Thirty five adult patients with acute leukaemia, first diagnosed or in relapse, who were admitted to our hospital between 30 November 1981 and 1 November 1983, were randomized to a group receiving colistin plus neomycin or to a group receiving colistin plus trimethoprim-sulfamethoxazole. Colistin (200 mg) and neomycin (250 mg) were given every 6 h and trimethoprim (240 mg)-sulfamethoxazole (1200 mg) every 12 hours. All patients received antifungal prophylaxis with amphotericin B tablets (200 mg) plus amphotericin B (200 mg) or nystatin (1×10^6 U) suspension every 6 hours. No measures for protective isolation were taken. For ANLL the antileukaemic treatment consisted of a combination of thioguanine, cytosine arabinoside and daunorubicin (14); sometimes doxorubicin, vincristine and an intermediate dose cytosine arabinoside was used (15). The patients with ALL were treated according to a Dutch protocol for ALL, which consisted of six weekly doses of vincristine and daily prednisone with daunorubicin (60 mg/m^2) during three days in the second week of induction therapy. During this period three intrathecal injections with methotrexate (15 mg) were given (16). The indications for parenteral antibiotics and the clinical investigations were the same as described previously (7,17). Surveillance cultures were obtained from the throat, urine and faeces at time of admission and thereafter at least once weekly. The microbiological methods used to isolate and identify bacteria were the same as described previously (7), except that anaerobic stool cultures were not done. Patients who either were older than 65 years or were known to be allergic for trimethoprim-sulfamethoxazole were not included in this study. Five patients were considered as nonevalua-

Table 1. Clinical data from patients with acute leukaemia

	Colistin + neomycin	Colistin + trimethoprim-sulfamethoxazole
Patients (n)	15	15
Mean age (yrs)	41	37
Patients infected at admission (n)	2	4
First induction remission (n)	9	12
Acute nonlymphocytic leukaemia (n)	12	11
Antileukaemic courses (mean) (n)	1.8	2
Complete remissions (n)	11	11
Partial remissions (n)	3	2
Granulocyte count 101 to 499/μl (mean) (d)	9.6	8.3
Granulocyte count < 100/μl (mean ± SD) (d)	31.1 ± 11.4	31.9 ± 10.7
associated with fever (%)	35*	24*
Parenteral antibiotics during granulocytopenic periods (% of days)	50	28

* Not significant with the two-sample test of Wilcoxon.

ble: four died in the first week of induction therapy and one patient developed a severe allergic reaction to trimethoprim-sulfamethoxazole and was excluded.

RESULTS

Thirty patients with acute leukaemia who received remission induction treatment could be evaluated. The clinical data of the patients are summarized in Table 1. The groups were similar with respect to age, type of leukaemia, first diagnosis or relapse and the duration of bone marrow aplasia caused by intensive cytotoxic regimens. No significant difference in the incidence of fever was observed. The use of parenteral antibiotics was lower in the group which received colistin plus trimethoprim-sulfamethoxazole.

Nine acquired infections (one major, eight minor) occurred in the group of patients who received CT versus fourteen infections (seven major, seven minor) in the other group (Table 2). The incidence of infections caused by gram-negative bacilli was low in both groups. A significant reduction of gram-positive infections (including mixed infections) was found in the patients treated with colistin plus trimethoprim-sulfamethoxazole ($p < 0.05$, $\chi^2 = 4.26$). Three local infections of the oropharynx caused by *Candida* were observed in the CT group versus two in the CN group. One disseminated candida infection and one aspergillus infection were observed in the CN group.

Table 2. Microbiological documentation of acquired infections

	Colistin + neomycin	Colistin + trimethoprim-sulfamethoxazole
Patients (n)	15	15
Acquired infections* (n)	14	9
Patients without acquired infections	3	7
Clinically documented infections	5	6
Bacteriologically documented infections	9 (6)	3 (1)
gram-positive bacteria**	6 (3)	1
Staphylococcus aureus	3	1
Staphylococcus epidermidis	1 (1)	-
Streptococcus	2 (2)	-
gram-negative bacteria	2 (2)	2 (1)
Escherichia coli	-	-
Klebsiella	-	1 (1)
Pseudomonas aeruginosa	1 (1)	-
Acinetobacter	-	1
Haemophilus influenzae	1 (1)	-
gram-positive and gram-negative bacteria	1 (1)	-
E. coli + Streptococcus		

* Not including infections caused by yeasts or fungi.
** $p < 0.05$, $\chi^2 = 4.26$.
Parentheses indicate number of cases with bacteraemia.

No difference was found with respect to the site of infections. In the group of patients not receiving trimethoprim-sulfamethoxazole more episodes of septicaemias were seen, defined as an episode with fever and a positive blood culture whereby no site of infection was found (Table 3).

In the surveillance cultures obtained from one week after the onset of selective decontamination, resistant gram-negative microorganisms were isolated from about half of the patients (Table 4). However, the colonization rate with resistant microorganisms was low: in five patients from the CN group (two strains of the oropharynx and three strains of the lower alimentary tract) and in one patient from the CT group (oropharynx). Only in the last patient colonization with trimethoprim- sulfamethoxazole resistant *Enterobacteriaceae* was followed by an infection. *Proteus spp.* were more often recovered from the surveillance cultures of the CN group because these strains are usually sensitive to trimethoprim-sulfamethoxazole and not to colistin and neomycin. In one patient septicaemia with *Pseudomonas* sensitive to colistin occurred without any evidence of these bacteria in previous surveillance cultures.

Four patients in the CT group developed an allergic reaction probably due to the sulfa component; three patients could be further treated with the combination of colistin and trimethoprim. No allergic reactions were observed in the patients receiving colistin plus neomycin.

Table 3. Sites of infection

Infection	Colistin + neomycin	Colistin + trimethoprim-sulfamethoxazole
Pneumonia	1*	0
Upper respiratory tract	0	2
Oropharynx	4	4 (1)
Anorectal	0	0
Urinary tract	0	0
Skin and soft tissue	3	2
No site found ('septicaemia')	6**	0**
Miscellaneous	0	1
Total	14	9

* One pneumonia caused by *Aspergillus* not included.
** $p < 0.05$, $\chi^2 = 5.20$.

Table 4. The prevalence of resistant gram-negative bacilli

	Colistin + neomycin	Colistin + trimethoprim-sulfamethoxazole
Patients (n)	15	15
Transient* microorganisms/patients	9/7 (0)	9/8 (0)
Escherichia coli	2	1
Citrobacter	–	1
Klebsiella	–	–
Enterobacter	0	4
Proteus	3	–
Pseudomonas	2	1
Acinetobacter	2	2
Colonizing** microorganisms/patients	5/5 (0)	1/1 (1)
Escherichia coli	1	–
Klebsiella	–	1 (1)
Enterobacter	1	–
Proteus	3	–
Pseudomonas	–	–
Acinetobacter	–	–

* Microorganisms appearing in one single culture.
** Microorganisms appearing in consecutive cultures.
Resistant microorganisms: resistant to trimethoprim-sulfamethoxazole and/or neomycin and/or to colistin.
Parentheses indicate number of cases with subsequent infection.

DISCUSSION

In this study two regimens were used for infection prevention in patients with acute leukaemia: one with only nonabsorbable drugs (colistin plus neomycin) and one using nonabsorbable plus absorbable drugs (colistin plus trimethoprim-sulfamethoxazole). The results show that both regimens are similarly effective in preventing infections caused by aerobic gram-negative microorganisms. Colonization of the alimentary tract with potential pathogens occurred only in a few cases. The appearance of *Proteus spp.* in patients receiving colistin with neomycin is not surprising because these microorganisms are not sensitive to colistin. This is not necessarily a disadvantage of this regimen because colonization with *Proteus* is rarely followed by a subsequent infection (18-20). The low incidence of colonization of the oropharynx in both groups supports the idea that the gut flora and the oropharyngeal flora are closely related (21-23), and that the intestines are the most likely reservoir for these microorganisms (23). Selective decontamination of the microbial flora of the gut seems to be the most important way to prevent colonization of the oropharynx. For this purpose a systemic antibiotic effect, e.g. trimethoprim-sulfamethoxazole, is not needed. A favourable effect of selective decontamination on the oropharyngeal flora may result in a decrease of bacterial pneumonia (24-26). However one should be aware of a relative increase in pneumonia caused by *Aspergillus spp.* (6,9). In the total number of 86 patients (this study and the patients described in the two previous chapters) who received selective decontamination we have observed eight acquired pneumonias three of which were caused by *Aspergillus spp.*

The addition of systemic antibiotics such as trimethoprim-sulfamethoxazole reduced the number of infections caused by gram-positive bacteria ($p < 0.05$), confirming our previous findings (7,17). There was a lower incidence of septicaemias in the group of patients treated with colistin plus trimethoprim-sulfamethoxazole: no episodes of septicaemias were seen compared to six in the CN group ($p < 0.05$).

The efficacy of trimethoprim-sulfamethoxazole alone for infection prevention has been confirmed in a large number of studies (5-7,9,27-31). A serious drawback of the use of trimethoprim-sulfamethoxazole alone can be the emergence of resistant microorganisms (6,7,9,30,32) although this was not observed by other investigators (27,29,31,33,34). The prevalence of resistance to this agent in the hospital environment combined with opportunities for cross-infection probably plays an important role (35). This study confirms our previous experience (17) that selective decontamination with a combination of drugs, e.g. colistin plus trimethoprim-sulfamethoxazole or colistin plus neomycin, prevents colonization with resistant gram- negative microorganisms in nearly all patients.

Four patients developed allergic reactions to trimethoprim-sulfamethoxazole, especially to the sulfa component, three of them could be treated further with trimethoprim.

The duration of granulocytopenia was not different between the two groups of patients. The prolonged and profound granulocytopenia in all patients reflects the intensive remission induction treatment which was used. No evidence of bone marrow suppression was found in the patients treated with trimethoprim-sulfamethoxazole, contrary to our previous study (7,36) and other studies (9,37) using the same doses. Possibly the delay in granulocyte recovery is dose dependent (38). Authors who have used lower doses of trimethoprim-sulfamethoxazole did not find any influence (6,27-31,39). It might be that the more intensive cytotoxic therapy used in this study as compared with the previous one has obscured a possible delay in bone marrow recovery caused by trimethoprim- sulfamethoxazole.

In conclusion this study shows that both regimens were effective in prevention of infections caused by aerobic gram-negative bacilli. Colonization with resistant microorganisms can be prevented in most cases. We prefer to use the combination of colistin plus trimethoprim-sulfamethoxazole because the systemic activity of the last drug seems to decrease the occurrence of infections and septicaemias caused by gram-positive bacteria.

REFERENCES

1. Van der Waaij D, Berghuis-de Vries JM, Lekkerkerk-van der Wees JEC. Colonization resistance of the digestive tract in conventional and antibiotic-treated mice. J Hyg (Camb) 69: 405-411, 1971.
2. Van der Waaij D, Berghuis-de Vries JM. Selective elimination of Enterobacteriaceae species from the digestive tract in mice and monkeys. J Hyg (Camb) 72: 205-211, 1974.
3. Guiot HFL, van Furth R. Partial antibiotic decontamination. Br Med J 1: 800-802, 1977.
4. Guiot HFL, van der Meer JWM, van Furth R. Selective antimicrobial modulation of human microbial flora: Infection prevention in patients with decreased host defense mechanisms by selective elimination of potentially pathogenic bacteria. J Infect Dis 143: 644-644, 1981.
5. Sleijfer DTh, Mulder NH, de Vries-Hospers HG, Fidler V, Nieweg HO, van der Waaij D, van Saene HKF. Infection prevention in granulocytopenic patients by selective decontamination of the digestive tract. Eur J Cancer 16: 859-869, 1980.
6. Wade JC, Schimpff SC, Hargadon MT, Fortner CL, Young VM, Wiernik PH. A comparison of trimethoprim-sulfamethoxazole plus nystatin with gentamicin plus nystatin in the prevention of infections in acute leukemia. New Engl J Med 304: 1057-1062, 1981.
7. Dekker AW, Rozenberg-Arska M, Sixma JJ, Verhoef J. Prevention of infection by trimethoprim-sulfamethoxazole plus amphotericin B in patients with acute nonlymphocytic leukaemia. Ann Intern Med 95: 555-559, 1981.
8. Guiot HFL, van den Broek PJ, van der Meer JWM, van Furth R. Selective antimicrobial modulation of the intestinal flora of patients with acute nonlymphocytic leukemia: A double-blind, placebo-controlled study. J Infect Dis 147: 615-623, 1983.
9. Wade JC, de Jongh CA, Newman KA, Crowley J, Wiernik PH, Schimpff SC. Selective

antimicrobial modulation as prophylaxis against infection during granulocytopenia: trimethoprim-sulfamethoxazole vs. nalidixic acid. J Infect Dis 147: 624-634, 1983.
10. Van der Waaij D. Colonization resistance of the digestive tract as a major lead in the selection of antibiotics for therapy. In: New Criteria for Antimicrobial Therapy: Maintenance of Digestive Tract Colonization Resistance. Proceedings of a Symposium, Utrecht, January 1979. Van der Waaij D, Verhoef J (eds), Excerpta Medica, Amsterdam-Oxford, pp 271-282, 1979.
11. Wiegersma N, Jansen G, van der Waaij D. Effect of twelve antimicrobial drugs on the colonization resistance of the digestive tract of mice and on endogenous potentially pathogenic bacteria. J Hyg (Camb) 88: 221-230, 1982.
12. Van der Waaij D, Aberson J, Thijm HA, Welling GW. The screening of four aminoglycosides in the selective decontamination of the digestive tract in mice. Infection 10: 43-48, 1982.
13. E.O.R.T.C. Gnotobiotic Project Group. Protocol for a prospective randomized study on the comparison of two regimens of selective decontamination for the prevention of infection in acute leukaemia patients. October 1981.
14. Gale RP, Foon KA, Cline MJ, Zighelboim J, The UCLA Acute Leukaemia Study Group. Intensive chemotherapy for acute myelogenous leukemia. Ann Intern Med 94: 753-757, 1981.
15. Van Prooijen HC, Dekker AW, Punt K. The use of intermediate dose cytosine arabinoside (ID Ara-C) in the treatment of acute non-lymphocytic leukaemia in relapse. Br J Haematol (in press), 1984.
16. HOVON. Protocol ALL, May 1982.
17. Rozenberg-Arska M, Dekker AW, Verhoef J. Colistin and trimethoprim-sulfamethoxazole for the prevention of infection in patients with acute non-lymphocytic leukaemia. Decrease in the emergence of resistant bacteria. Infection 11: 167-169, 1983.
18. Bodey GP, Rodriguez V, Chang H-Y, Narboni G. Fever and infection in leukemic patients. Cancer 41: 1610-1622, 1978.
19. Newman KA, Schimpff SC, Young VM, Wiernik PH. Lessons learned from surveillance cultures in patients with acute nonlymphocytic leukemia. Am J Med 70: 423-431, 1981.
20. Cohen ML, Murphy MT, Counts GW, Buckner CD, Clift RA, Meyers JD. Prediction by surveillance cultures of bacteremia among neutropenic patients treated in a protective environment. J Infect Dis 147: 789-793, 1983.
21. LeFrock JL, Ellis CA, Weinstein L. The impact of hospitalization on the aerobic fecal microflora. Am J Med Sci 277: 269-274, 1979.
22. LeFrock JL, Ellis CA, Weinstein L. The relation between aerobic fecal and oropharyngeal microflora in hospitalized patients. Am J Med Sci 277: 275-280, 1979.
23. Fainstein V, Rodriguez V, Turck M, Hermann G, Rosenbaum B, Bodey GP. Patterns of oropharyngeal and fecal flora in patients with acute leukemia. J Infect Dis 144: 10-18, 1981.
24. Johanson WG, Pierce AK, Sandford YP, Thomas GD. Nosocomial respiratory infections with gram-negative bacilli. Ann Intern Med 77: 701-706, 1972.
25. Huxley EJ, Viroslav J, Gray WR, Pierce AK. Pharyngeal aspiration in normal adults and patients with depressed consiousness. Am J Med 64: 564-568, 1978.
26. Eickhoff TC. Nosocomial respiratory tract infections: the gastrointestinal tract as a reservoir. In: New Criteria for Antimicrobial Therapy: Maintenance of Digestive Tract Colonization Resistance. Van der Waaij D, Verhoef J (eds). Excerpta Medica, Amsterdam-Oxford, pp 5-11, 1979.
27. Gurwith MJ, Brunton JI, Lank BA, Harding GKM, Ronald AR. A prospective

controlled investigation of prophylactic trimethoprim/sulfamethoxazole in hospitalized granulocytopenic patients. Am J Med 66: 248-256, 1979.

28. Starke ID, Catovsky D, Johnson SA, Donelly P, Darrell J, Goldman JM, Galton DAG. Co-trimoxazole alone for prevention of bacterial infection in patients with acute leukaemia. The Lancet i: 5-6, 1982.
29. Watson JG, Powles RL, Lawson DM, Morgenstern GR, Jameson B, McElwain TM, Judson I, Lumley H, Kay HEM. Co-trimoxazole versus non-absorbable antibiotics in acute leukaemia. The Lancet i: 6-9, 1982.
30. Gualtieri RJ, Donowitz GR, Kaiser DL, Hess CE, Sande MA. Double-blind randomized study of prophylactic trimethoprim/sulfamethoxazole in granulocytopenic patients with hematologic malignancies. Am J Med 74: 934-940, 1983.
31. Kauffman CA, Leipman MK, Bergman AG, Mioduszewski J. Trimethoprim/sulfamethoxazole prophylaxis in neutropenic patients. Reduction of infections and effect on bacterial and fungal flora. Am J Med 74: 599-607, 1983.
32. Wilson JM, Guiney DG. Failure of oral trimethoprim-sulfamethoxazole prophylaxis in acute leukemia. New Engl J Med 306: 16-20, 1982.
33. De Vries-Hospers HG. Selective decontamination of the digestive tract in granulocytopenic patients; the occurrence of resistance. In: New Criteria for Antimicrobial Therapy: Maintenance of Digestive Tract Colonization Resistance. Proceedings of a Symposium, Utrecht, January 1979. Van der Waaij D, Verhoef J (eds). Excerpta Medica, Amsterdam-Oxford, pp 117-129, 1979.
34. Weiser B, Lange M, Fialk MA, Singer C, Szatrowski TH, Armstrong D. Prophylactic trimethoprim-sulfamethoxazole during consolidation chemotherapy for acute leukemia: A controlled trial. Ann Intern Med 95: 436-438, 1981.
35. Young LS. Antimicrobial prophylaxis against infection in neutropenic patients. J Infect Dis 147: 611-614, 1983.
36. Dekker AW, Rozenberg-Arska M, Sixma JJ, Verhoef J. In response to a letter to the editor: Trimethoprim-sulfamethoxazole and granulocytopenia. Ann Intern Med 96: 381-382, 1982.
37. Pizzo PA, Robichaud KJ, Edwards BK, Schumaker C, Kramer BS, Johnson A. Oral antibiotic prophylaxis in patient with cancer: A double-blind randomized placebo-controlled trial. J Pediat 102: 125-133, 1983.
38. Deeg HJ, Meyers JD, Storb R, Graham TC, Weiden PL. Effect of trimethoprim-sulfamethoxazole on hematological recovery after total body irradiation and autologous marrow infusion in dogs. Transplantation 28: 243-246, 1979.
39. Enno A, Darrell J, Hows J, Catovsky D, Goldman JM, Galton DAG. Co-trimoxazole for prevention of infection in acute leukaemia. Lancet i: 395-397, 1978.

CHAPTER 8

General discussion

Acute nonlymphocytic leukaemia is for many of the patients still an incurable disease with a poor longterm prognosis. Only after achievement of complete remission a prolongation of survival and a chance of cure can be expected. Until the end of 1981 we obtained with our at the time commonly used remission induction therapy a complete remission rate of about 50 percent; 66 percent in patients younger than 50 years and 29 percent in older patients. The results were similar to recent studies using comparable remission induction regimens (1,2,3). We now apply more intensive schedules (4) to improve these results. An important number of patients, however, does not achieve a remission and expires within a few months. An optimal supportive care and institute experience is mandatory in the treatment of patients with acute leukaemia otherwise many will not survive the toxic effects of such more intensive schedules. Especially elderly patients are highly susceptible to complications of bone marrow hypoplasia and to the side effects of chemotherapy.

In our study we found an increase in early death in promyelocytic leukaemia and hyperleucocytosis. Another approach in these patients is necessary. In patients with hyperleucocytosis reduction of the leukaemic cell mass by leukapheresis reverses the hyperleucocytic syndrome rapidly and prevents the risk of cytolysis induced metabolic changes (5,6,7,8). A recent study shows that leukapheresis as initial treatment of patients with hyperleucocytosis improves the remission induction rate (9). Several studies using heparin with intensive platelet transfusions in the induction remission phase of promyelocytic leukaemia suggest that this approach may decrease early death due to bleeding (10-12). Our experience is different: three out of six patients with promyelocytic leukaemia treated in this way died during the first week of therapy due to cerebral bleeding. Therefore the use of low molecular weight fractions of heparin with a high anti-Xa activity but little effect on thrombin, combined with platelet transfusions, seems more appropriate for the management of symptomatic diffuse intravascular coagulation in promyelocytic leukaemia (13,14), because these fractions cause less bleeding and possess the same antithrombotic effect. A cooperative pilot study about this is currently in progress.

We have not studied the predictive value of some properties of the leukaemic cells such as chromosomal karyotypes, in vitro growth patterns or sensitivity to cytotoxic agents. Previous findings showing that an abnormal karyotype is an unfavourable prognostic factor (15,16) could not be confirmed by more recent data (17,18). The introduction of more effective chemotherapy may have lessened the influence of a clonal chromosome abnormality as a prognostic factor (19). Because in vitro clonogenic culture techniques for leukaemic cells are difficult to perform only a few studies are available; limited leukaemic cell growth in vitro seems to be associated with a higher response rate (20-22). More promising are studies on the in vitro sensitivity of clonogenic leukaemic cells to cytotoxic agents, especially to cytosine arabinoside (23-25). Although the number of patients with resistant disease is rather low, approximately 10-15 percent (26), early recognition of drug resistant disease may be of value. Easier methods to determine drug resistant disease are the bone marrow cellularity at the end of the first course (27) or the percentage of residual leukaemic cells just before the second course of chemotherapy (28).

Increase of the remission rate alone, however, is not sufficient for improvement of the prospects of patients with acute nonlymphocytic leukaemia. The median duration of remission in our study was only eight months despite the use of maintenance chemotherapy, and continuous remissions were rare. An explanation for these results might be the at the time common practice of using relatively low doses of cytotoxic drugs during remission induction treatment not followed by an intensive consolidation regimen. In most cases the bone marrow was the first site of relapse. The chance to achieve a second remission depends on the maintenance therapy used before. A second remission rate of about 50 percent has been reported (29) and was also achieved in our group of patients. Although we even obtained a high third remission rate (30), the outlook on a longterm survival after a relapse remains poor and nearly all patients die within one year after the first relapse (31).

We have observed a relatively high incidence of symptomatic meningeal leukaemia: nine cases out of 46 patients with a complete response (20 percent). Also after exclusion of three patients with a prior bone marrow relapse the occurrence of meningeal leukaemia remained considerable high (13 percent). A possible factor contributing to this high incidence might be the less intensive cytotoxic regimen we have used. We found that patients with extramedullary involvement at initial diagnosis and probably also patients with hyperleucocytosis had an increased risk of meningeal leukaemia. A more rapid achievement of remission may decrease the occurrence of meningeal leukaemia because leukaemic cells invade the leptomeninges probably by the time of initial haematological diagnosis or shortly thereafter. Central nervous system prophylaxis in acute nonlymphocytic leukaemia does not prolong the duration of remission or survival (4). However, in order to prevent the severe morbidity of meningeal leukaemia prophylactic measures are indicated: a diagnostic lumbar puncture after the achievement of remission in all patients for early treatment in case of asymptomatic meningeal leukaemia, and intrathecal prophylaxis with cytosine arabinoside for the subgroup of patients at higher risk.

More intensive remission induction- and post- remission induction chemotherapy does improve not only the remission rate (to 70-80 percent) but also the median duration of remission (to 12-14 months) while a proportion of patients remain in continuous remission (10-20 percent). The changes of longterm survival remain poor with this approach for the majority of patients. At present, the only chance of improving the rate of cure or of longterm survival seems to be intensification of post-remission induction treatment. Other approaches such as different forms of immunotherapy are of no substantial benefit in prolonging the duration of remission or survival (4,32-34). The most promising type of intensive post- remission induction therapy is high dose cyclophosphamide with (35) or without (36) total body irradiation and followed by allogeneic bone marrow transplantation. The current results indicate that prolonged survival (and possibly cure) can be achieved in approximately 50 percent of patients younger than 40 years, who are in complete remission and have an HLA- identical sibling (35,37-43). Drawbacks of allogeneic bone marrow transplantation are the scarcity of suitable donors and the high incidence of early death due to infection, interstitial pneumonia or graft-versus-host disease (44). Autologous bone marrow transplantation avoids most of these problems and may permit the application of high dose chemotherapy and total body irradiation to eliminate residual leukaemia. However, as long as no successful techniques are available to separate normal from leukaemic cells, autologous bone marrow cells remain contaminated with leukaemic cells. As could be expected the results of autologous bone marrow transplantation in patients in relapse are not hopeful (45-48), more promising is this approach for patients during the first remission (49-51). Autologous bone marrow transplantation should be regarded as an alternative form of post-remission induction chemotherapy aiming at the prolongation of disease-free survival.

A prerequisite for the use of more intensive cytotoxic chemotherapy is optimal supportive care. Infection is still a common cause of death during bone marrow hypoplasia. Many infections are caused by microorganisms that normally colonize the alimentary tract. Selective decontamination, by the use of certain antimicrobial agents, eliminates potential pathogenic microorganisms and may be a promising approach for the prevention of infections caused by aerobic gram-negative bacilli. If that is true, complicated and expensive isolation measures are not needed. We investigated several antimicrobial regimens for selective decontamination: trimethoprim-sulfamethoxazole, colistin plus trimethoprim-sulfamethoxazole, and colistin plus neomycin. A significant decrease of more that 50 percent of acquired infections caused by gram-negative microorganisms was observed. However, in our opinion the use of trimethoprim-sulfamethoxazole alone is not advisable because we found a high rate of colonization and subsequent infection by resistant gram-negative bacilli. The best results were obtained with a combination of trimethoprim-sulfamethoxazole and colistin. The addition of colistin to trimethoprim- sulfamethoxazole prevented colonization of the lower alimentary tract with resistant gram-negative bacilli, but trimethoprim-sulfamethoxazole resistant microorganisms may be isolated from the oropharynx because colistin tablets do not have a direct effect on the upper alimentary tract. No colistin resistant strains were recovered from surveillance cultures except for *Proteus spp.* which are known to be insensitive to colistin. In addition to a selective decontaminating effect of trimethoprim-sulfamethoxazole this drug also decreased the incidence of infections and septicaemias caused by gram-positive bacteria. Other investigators (52-54) also observed this favourable effect which is probably caused by the systemic activity of this drug.

One should be aware of trimethoprim-sulfamethoxazole resistant viridans streptococci (55) or *Staphylococcus epidermidis* infections (56). Prophylactic antibiotic regimens may promote colonization with *Staphylococcus epidermidis* and may lead to an increased incidence of bacteraemia with these microorganisms (57). Prolonged hospitalization, profound granulocytopenia, parenteral hyperalimentation and intravascular catheters are also predisposing factors (58). The surveillance cultures from the oropharyngeal and faecal flora were helpful in predicting infections caused by *Enterobacteriaceae*, but not infections caused by *Pseudomonas* which occurred mostly without previous evidence of these bacteria in these surveillance cultures. The incidence of infections caused by *Pseudomonas* was found to be rather low, however, and therefore had not changed our first choice of therapeutical antibiotic treatment. There was no evidence that the response to parenteral antibiotic therapy was different in patients with or without a prophylactic regimen. The use of antifungal prophylaxis during selective decontamination did not always prevent localized infections of the upper alimentary tract caused by *Candida* (in fourteen percent of the patients). Severe candidal infections, however, were rare although the detection of disseminated candidiasis is difficult and remains primarily a clinical diagnosis (59). Antifungal prophylaxis does not protect against infections caused by *Aspergillus spp.* and a relative increase in invasive aspergillosis may occur. One should suspect pulmonary aspergillosis when a patient with pneumonia does not respond to antibiotic therapy. This is important because the outcome of invasive aspergillosis correlates directly with early diagnosis and therapy (60,61).

The combination of colistin and trimethoprim-sulfamethoxazole is an effective regimen for the prevention of infections in patients with prolonged and profound granulocytopenia. However, it may have some drawbacks: the large number of tablets to be taken, possible delay in granulocyte recovery and an increasing number of allergic reactions. Promising alternatives, which are now under investigation, are the new nalidixic acid derivates such as ciprofloxacin and norfloxacin, which also have a potent activity against *Pseudomonas* and gram-positive cocci including *Staphylococcus epidermidis* (62,63). These highly active antibacterial agents may be suitable for selective decontamination.

REFERENCES

1. Keating MJ, Smith TL, McCredie KB, Bodey GP, Hersh EM, Gutterman JU, Gehan E, Freireich EJ. A four-year experience with anthracycline, cytosine arabinoside, vincristine and prednisone combination chemotherapy in 325 adults with acute leukemia. Cancer 47: 2779-2788, 1981.
2. McCredie KB, Gehan EA, Freireich EJ, Hewlett JS, Coltman CA, Hussein KK, Balcerzak SP, Chen TT. Management of adult acute leukemia. A southwest oncology group study. Cancer 52: 958-966, 1983.
3. Lister TA, Whitehouse JMA, Oliver RTD, Bell R, Johnson SAN, Wrigley PFM, Ford JM, Cullen MH, Gregory W, Paxton AM, Malpas JS. Chemotherapy and immunotherapy for acute myelogenous leukemia. Cancer 46: 2142-2148, 1980.
4. Gale RP, Foon KA, Cline MJ, Zighelboim J, and the UCLA acute leukemia study group. Intensive chemotherapy for acute myelogenous leukemia. Ann Intern Med 94: 753-757, 1981.
5. Eisenstaedt RS, Berkman EM. Rapid cytoreduction in acute leukemia. Management of cerebral leukostasis by cell pheresis. Transfusion 18: 113-115, 1978.
6. Lane TA. Continuous-flow leukapheresis for rapid cytoreduction in leukemia. Transfusion 20: 455-457, 1980.
7. Karp DD, Beck JR, Cornell Jr CJ. Chronic granulocytic leukemia with respiratory distress. Arch Intern Med 141: 1353-1354, 1981.
8. Lichtman MA, Rowe JM. Hyperleukocytic leukemias: Rheological, clinical and therapeutic considerations. Blood 60: 279-283, 1982.
9. Cuttner J, Holland JF, Norton L, Ambinder E, Button G, Meyer RJ. Therapeutic leukapheresis for hyperleukocytosis in acute myelocytic leukemia. Med Pediat Oncol 11: 76-78, 1983.
10. Drapkin RL, Gee TS, Dowling MD, Arlin Z, McKenzie S, Kempin S, Clarkson B. Prophylactic heparin therapy in acute promyelocytic leukemia. Cancer 41: 2484-2490, 1978.
11. Collins AJ, Bloomfield CD, Peterson BA, McKenna RW, Edson R. Acute promyelocytic leukemia. Management of the coagulopathy during daunorubicin- prednisone remission induction. Arch Intern Med 138: 1677-1680, 1978.
12. Sandler RM, Liebman HA, Patch MJ, Teitelbaum A, Levine AM, Feinstein DI.

Antithrombin III and anti- activated factor X activity in patients with acute promyelocytic leukemia and disseminated intravascular coagulation treated with heparin. Cancer 51: 681-685, 1983.
13. Andersson L-O, Barrowcliffe TW, Holmer E, Johnson EA, Sims GEC. Anticoagulant properties of heparin fractionated by affinity chromatography on matrix-bound antithrombin III and by gel filtration. Thromb Res 9: 575-583, 1976.
14. Kakkar VV, Djazaeri B, Fok J, Fletcher M, Scully MF, Westwick J. Low-molecular-weight heparin and prevention of postoperative deep vein thrombosis. Br Med J 284: 375-379, 1982.
15. Golomb HM, Vardiman J, Rowley JD. Acute nonlymphocytic leukemia in adults: correlations with Q-banded chromosomes. Blood 48: 9-21, 1976.
16. Golomb HM, Vardiman JW, Rowley JD, Testa JR, Mintz U. Correlation of clinical findings with quinacrine- banded chromosomes in 90 adults with acute nonlymphocytic leukemia. An eight-year study (1970-1977). New Engl J Med 299: 613-619, 1978.
17. Li YS, Khalid G, Hayhoe FGJ. Correlation between chromosomal pattern, cytological subtypes, response to therapy and survival in acute myeloid leukaemia. Scand J Haematol 30: 265-277, 1983.
18. Brodeur GM, Williams DL, Kalwinsky DK, Williams KJ, Dahl GV. Cytogenetic features of acute nonlymphoblastic leukemia in 73 children and adolescents. Cancer Genet Cytogenet 8: 93-105, 1983.
19. Bloomfield CD, Arthur DC. Evaluation of leukemic-cell chromosomes as a guide to therapy. Blood cells 8: 501-518, 1982.
20. Spitzer G, Dicke KA, Gehan EA, Smith T, McCredie KB, Barlogie B, Freireich EJ. A simplified in vitro classification for prognosis in adult acute leukemia: the application of in vitro results in remission-predictive models. Blood 48: 795-807, 1976.
21. Vincent PC, Sutherland R, Bradley M, Lind D, Gunz FW. Marrow culture studies in adult acute leukemia at presentation and during remission. Blood 49: 903-912, 1977.
22. Beran M, Reizenstein P, Uden A-M. Response to treatment in acute non-lymphatic leukaemia: prognostic value of colony forming and colony stimulating capacities of bone marrow and blood cells compared to other parameters. Br J Haematol 44: 39-50, 1980.
23. Preisler HD. Prediction of response to chemotherapy in acute myelocytic leukemia. Blood 56: 361-367, 1980.
24. McCulloch EA, Curtis JE, Messner HA, Senn JS, Germanson TP. The contribution of blast cell properties to outcome variation in acute myeloblastic leukemia (AML). Blood 59: 601-608, 1982.
25. Marie J-P, Zittoun R, Thevenin D, Mathieu M, Viguie F. In vitro culture of clonogenic leukaemic cells in acute myeloid leukaemia: growth pattern and drug sensitivity. Br J Haematol 55: 427-437, 1983.
26. Preisler HD. Treatment failure in AML. Blood Cells 8: 585-602, 1982.
27. Preisler H, Barcos M, Reese P, Priore RL, Pothier L. Recognition of drug resistance during remission induction therapy for acute non-lymphocytic leukemia: utility of day 6 bone marrow biopsy. Leuk Res 7: 67-75, 1983.
28. Hasbrouck DJ, Peterson BA, Hurd DD, Bloomfield CD. Management of patients with acute non-lymphocytic leukemia who fail first cycle of induction therapy. Leuk Res 5: 357-361, 1981.
29. Peterson BA, Bloomfield CD. Re-induction of complete remissions in adults with acute non-lymphocytic leukemia. Leuk Res 5: 81-88, 1981.
30. Van Prooijen HC, Dekker AW, Punt K. The use of intermediate dose cytosine arabinoside (ID Ara-C) in the treatment of acute nonlymphocytic leukaemia in relapse. Br J Haematol 1984 (in press).
31. Glucksberg H, Cheever MA, Farewell VT, Fefer A, Sale GE, Thomas ED. High-dose

combination chemotherapy for acute nonlymphoblastic leukemia in adults. Cancer 48: 1073-1081, 1981.
32. Vogler WR. Results of randomized trials of immunotherapy for acute leukemia. Cancer Immunol Immunother 9: 15-21, 1980.
33. Baker MA, Taub RN, Carter WH, the Toronto leukemia study group. Immunotherapy for remission maintenance in acute myeloblastic leukemia. Cancer Immunol Immunother 13: 85-88, 1982.
34. Foon KA, Smalley RV, Riggs CW, Gale RP. The role of immunotherapy in acute myelogenous leukemia. Arch Intern Med 143: 1726-1731, 1983.
35. Thomas ED, Buckner CD, Clift RA, Fefer A, Johnson FL, Neiman PE, Sale GE, Sander JE, Singer JW, Shulman H, Storb R, Weiden PL. Marrow transplantation for acute nonlymphocytic leukemia in first remission. New Engl J Med 301: 597-599, 1979.
36. Santos GW, Tutschka PJ, Brookmeyer R, Saral R, Beschorner WE, Bias WB, Braine HG, Burns WH, Elfenbein GJ, Kaizer H, Mellits D, Sensenbrenner LL, Stuart RK, Yeager AM. Marrow transplantation for acute nonlymphocytic leukemia after treatment with busulfan and cyclophosphamide. New Engl J Med 309: 1347-1353, 1983.
37. Blume KG, Beutler E, Bross KJ, Chillar RK, Ellington OB, Fahey JL, Farbstein MJ, Forman SJ, Schmidt GM, Scott EP, Spruce WE, Turner A, Wolf JL. Bone-marrow ablation and allogeneic marrow transplantation in acute leukemia. New Engl J Med 302: 1041-1046, 1980.
38. Powles RL, Morgenstern G, Clink HM, Hedley D, Bandini G, Lumley H, Watson JG, Lawson D, Spence D, Barrett A, Jameson B, Lawler S, Kay HEM, McElwain TJ. The place of bone-marrow transplantation in acute myelogenous leukaemia, Lancet i: 1047-1050, 1980.
39. Thomas ED, Clift RA, Buckner CD. Marrow transplantaton for patients with acute nonlymphoblastic leukemia who achieve a first remission. Cancer Treat Rep 66: 1463-1466, 1982.
40. Kersey JH, Ramsay NKC, Kim T, McGlave P, Krivit W, Levitt S, Filipovich A, Woods W, O'Leary M, Coccia P, Nesbit ME. Allogeneic bone marrow transplantation in acute nonlymphocytic leukemia: a pilot study. Blood 60: 400-403, 1982.
41. Gale RP, Kay HEM, Rimm AA, Bortin MM. Bone-marrow transplantation for acute leukaemia in first remission. Lancet ii: 1006-1008, 1982.
42. Prentice HG. A review of the current status and techniques of allogeneic bone marrow transplantation for treatment of leukaemia. J Clin Pathol 36: 1207-1214, 1983.
43. O'Reilly RJ. Review. Allogeneic bone marrow transplantation: current status and future directions. Blood 62: 941-964, 1983.
44. Bortin MM, Gale RP, Kay HEM, Rimm AA. Bone marrow transplantation for acute myelogenous leukemia. Factors associated with early mortality. JAMA 249: 1166-1175, 1983.
45. Dicke KA, Zander A, Spitzer G, Verma DS, Peters L, Vellekoop L, McCredie KB, Hester J. Autologous bone-marrow transplantation in relapsed adult acute leukaemia. Lancet i: 514-517, 1979.
46. Gorin NC, Najman A, Salmon Ch, Muller JY, Petit JC, David R, Stachowiak J, Marie FH, Parlier Y, Duhamel G. High dose combination chemotherapy (TACC) with and without autologous bone marrow transplantation for the treatment of acute leukaemia and other malignant diseases. Kinetics of recovery of haemopoiesis. A preliminary study of 12 cases. Eur J Cancer 15: 1113-1119, 1979.
47. Herve P, Rozenbaum A, Plouvier E, Flesch M, Cahn, J.Y., Farradji A, Bergerat JP, Adjizian JC, Pignon B. Autologous bone marrow transplantation in acute myeloid leukemia in relapse or in complete remission. Cancer Treat Rep 66: 1983-1985, 1982.
48. Zander AR, Vellekoop L, Dicke KA, Keating MJ, McCredie KB, Legha SS, Spitzer G,

Verma D, Bodey GP. High-dose AMSA and autologous bone marrow transplantation in relapsed acute leukemia. Cancer Treat Rep 66: 1991-1992, 1982.

49. Lowenberg B, Abels J, van Bekkum DW, Dzoljic G, Hendriks WDH, van der Poel J, Sizoo W, Sintnicolaas K, Wagemaker G. Transplantatie van autoloog beenmerg bij 3 patienten met acute myeloide leukemie in eerste remissie; eerste ervaringen met een nieuwe behandeling. Ned Tijdschr Geneesk 127: 1329-1332, 1983.
50. De Gast GC. Zijn er perspectieven voor patienten met acute leukemie door transplantatie van autoloog beenmerg? Ned Tijdschr Geneesk 127: 1342-1344, 1983.
51. Gorin NC. Perspectives in cancer research. Autologous bone marrow transplantation in hematological malignancies. Eur J Cancer Clin Oncol 20: 1-9, 1984.
52. Hughes WT, Kuhn S, Chaudhary S, Feldman S, Verzosa M, Aur RJA, Pratt Ch, George SL. Successful chemoprophylaxis for pneumocystis carinii pneumonitis. New Engl J Med 297: 1419-1426, 1977.
53. Watson JG, Jameson B, Powles RL, McElwain TJ, Lawson DN, Judson I, Morgenstern GR, Lumley H, Kay HEM. Co-trimoxazole versus non-absorbable antibiotics in acute leukaemia. Lancet i: 6-9, 1982.
54. Kauffman CA, Liepman MK, Bergman AG, Mioduszewski J. Trimethoprim/sulfamethoxazole prophylaxis in neutropenic patients. Reduction of infections and effect on bacterial and fungal flora. Am J Med 74: 599-607, 1983.
55. Cohen J, Donnelly JP, Worsley AM, Catovsky D, Goldman JM, Galton DAG. Septicaemia caused by viridans streptococci in neutropenic patients with leukaemia. Lancet ii: 1452-1454, 1983.
56. Lowly FD, Hammer SM. Staphylococcus epidermidis infections. Ann Intern Med 99: 834-839, 1983.
57. Wade JC, Schimpff SC, Newman KA, Wiernik PH. Staphylococcus epidermidis: an increasing cause of infection in patients with granulocytopenia. Ann Intern Med 97: 503-508, 1982.
58. Christensen GD, Bisno AL, Parisi JT, McLaughlin B, Hester MG, Luther RW. Nosocomial septicemia due to multiply antibiotic-resistant staphylococcus epidermidis. Ann Intern Med 96: 1-10, 1982.
59. Edwards JE, Lehrer RI, Stiehm ER, Fischer TJ, Young LS. Severe candidal infections. Clinical perspective, immune defense mechanisms, and current concepts of therapy. Ann Intern Med 89: 91-106, 1978.
60. Aisner J, Schimpff SC, Wiernik PH. Treatment of invasive aspergillosis: relation of early diagnosis and treatment to response. Ann Intern Med 86: 539-543, 1977.
61. Rinaldi MG. Invasive aspergillosis. Rev Infect Dis 5: 1061-1077, 1983.
62. Norfloxacin. Microbiology-Pharmacology-Clinical evaluation. Eur J Clin Microbiol 2, 1983.
63. Editorial. The Quinolones. Lancet i: 24-25, 1984.

Summary

This thesis deals with some important aspects of the clinical management of adult patients with acute nonlymphocytic leukaemia (ANLL). Only the achievement of a complete remission gives a chance of a prolonged symptom-free period. The use of intensive cytotoxic chemotherapy and optimal supportive care are prerequisites for an effective remission induction treatment. They are the subject of this study.

In Chapter 1 the principles and development of cytotoxic chemotherapy in acute nonlymphocytic leukaemia are described and the results of recent clinical trials are reviewed. The controversial aspects of commonly accepted prognostic factors and their relative importance are discussed in detail.

Chapter 2 contains a retrospective analysis of 114 consecutive patients with ANLL who were admitted to the University Hospital of Utrecht between February 1977 and December 1981. Seven out of ten patients with secondary leukaemia were given induction therapy, but no complete remission was obtained. A group of 89 evaluable patients was analyzed for response to remission induction therapy consisting of doxorubicin, vincristine and cytosine arabinoside. The complete remission rate in this group was 48 percent, 66 percent in patients under the age of 50 and 29 percent in older patients ($p < 0.001$). In addition to older age, hyperleucocytosis ($> 100 \times 10^9$ cells per liter) was also an unfavourable factor for achieving complete remission: $p < 0.01$. The remission rate was not different in the FAB subclasses (excluding M3 and M6 which groups were too small for conclusions) and was not influenced by hepato- and/or splenomegaly and by the presence or absence of infection at the time of admission. The remission rate was similar to that in other studies in which comparable remission induction regimens were used. The median duration of remission was eight months and continuous remissions were rare. The results are slightly inferior to those in other studies in which a median duration of remission of approximately 12 months and 10-15 percent continuous remissions were reported. An explanation for this discrepancy could be that at the time of our study our remission induction treatment was not followed by an intensive consolidation regimen. However, the median survival time for complete responders (20 months) was the same as reported by others. This can be attributed to our high second remission rate of 50 percent.

Chapter 3 deals with the clinical aspects of symptomatic meningeal leukaemia in ANLL. No such cases occurred during remission induction therapy. Nine cases (20 percent) were observed in 46 complete responders: either as the only site of relapse (three patients) or together with a first bone marrow relapse (three patients) or following a bone marrow relapse (three patients). Extramedullary involvement at initial diagnosis was an independent predictive factor ($p = 0.005$). Four out of eight patients treated for meningeal leukaemia reached remission. Because the morbidity of symptomatic meningeal leukaemia and the therapy related toxicity are high, prophylactic treatment should be given in patients with an increased risk of meningeal leukaemia.

The next three chapters of this thesis describe clinical studies dealing with one of the most important aspects of supportive care in ANLL: the prevention of infections during remission induction treatment.

In Chapter 4 general considerations about the possibilities for infection prevention are given. Selective decontamination of the gastrointestinal tract seems to be the most promising approach for infection prevention because the alimentary tract is an important reservoir of potential pathogens. Strict isolation procedures are not needed in that case.

Chapter 5 describes the results of a randomized trial to ascertain the effect of prophylactic oral trimethoprim-sulfamethoxazole on the rate of infection and of fever in patients with ANLL during remission induction treatment. A decrease in the total number of acquired infections was found: 16 infections in 26 patients given trimethoprim-sulfamethoxazole versus 31 infections in 26 patients in the control group ($p < 0.01$). A disturbing phenomenon, however, was the emergence of resistant microorganisms: six out of nine bacteriologically documented infections in the trimethoprim-sulfamethoxazole group were caused by colonizing resistant microorganisms compared to two out of 20 in the control group.

In Chapter 6 the value of the addition of colistin to trimethoprim-sulfamethoxazole is discussed. Thirty patients received this combination during induction treatment. This regimen was effective in the prevention of infections, moreover a significant decrease ($p < 0.001$) occurred in the acquisition of and infection by gram-negative bacilli which were resistant to trimethoprim-sulfamethoxazole. Only two patients were colonized with resistant strains and no subsequent infection was observed.

Chapter 7 deals with the results of a randomized study of 30 patients who took part in an EORTC Gnotobiotic Project Group study. The aim of this study was to compare the value of a combination of nonabsorbable drugs, colistin plus neomycin (CN), with a combination of nonabsorbable and absorbable drugs, colistin plus trimethoprim-sulfamethoxazole (CT) in infection prevention. Both regimens appeared to be similarly effective in preventing infections caused by aerobic gram-negative bacilli. However, trimethoprim- sulfamethoxazole reduced the number of infections caused by gram-positive bacteria (one infection without bacteraemia in the CT group versus seven infections with four bacteraemias in the CN group, $p < 0.05$). For this reason the CT combination is preferable to CN. Four patients in the CT group developed allergic reactions probably due to the sulfa component.

In Chapter 8 a general discussion about the most relevant results of the foregoing studies is given. The remission rate in ANLL may be improved further by more intensive remission induction therapy, and specific measures such as leukapheresis in patients with hyperleucocytosis and the use of low molecular weight fractions of heparin in patients with promyelocytic leukaemia may reduce the early death rate. The initial establishment of drug resistant disease may lead to effective adjustments of the drug schedule used for induction therapy. Selective decontamination with the combination of colistin plus trimethoprim- sulfamethoxazole was proven to be of value for infection prevention during remission induction therapy. However, this combination necessitates the intake of a large number of tablets and may cause allergic reactions. For these reasons other antimicrobial drugs such as quinolones are now under investigation. Improvement of the remission rate alone is not sufficient for a better long term prognosis. For this purpose an intensive post-remission induction therapy is needed. A limited number of patients may benefit from bone marrow ablative therapy followed by bone marrow transplantation (allogeneic and possibly autologous).

Bei Fragen zur Produktsicherheit wenden Sie sich bitte an:
If you have any questions regarding product safety,
please contact:

Walter de Gruyter GmbH
Genthiner Straße 13
10785 Berlin
productsafety@degruyterbrill.com